The Rough Guide to
Mindfulness

Credits

The Rough Guide to Mindfulness

Editing and layout: Matthew Milton
Posture diagrams: Mike Hall
Proofreading: Jason Freeman,
Susannah Wight
Production: Gemma Sharpe,
Charlotte Cade

Rough Guides Reference

Editors: Kate Berens, Tom Cabot,
Tracy Hopkins, Matthew Milton,
Joe Staines
Director: Andrew Lockett

Publishing Information

This first edition published January 2013 by
Rough Guides Ltd, 80 Strand, London WC2R 0RL
11 Community Centre, Panchsheel Park, New Delhi 110017, India
Email: mail@roughguides.com

Distributed by the Penguin Group:
Penguin Books Ltd, 80 Strand, London WC2R 0RL
Penguin Group (USA), 375 Hudson Street, NY 10014, USA
Penguin Group (Australia), 250 Camberwell Road, Camberwell, Victoria 3124, Australia
Penguin Group (New Zealand), 67 Apollo Drive, Rosedale, Auckland 0632, New Zealand

Rough Guides is represented in Canada by Tourmaline Editions Inc.,
662 King Street West, Suite 304, Toronto

Printed in Singapore by Toppan Security Printing Pte. Ltd.

The Rough Guide to
Mindfulness

by Albert Tobler
and Susann Herrmann

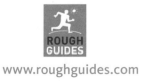

www.roughguides.com

Contents

Audio versions of the mindfulness exercises featured in this
book can be downloaded at **www.roughguides.com/mindfulness**

Acknowledgements

We wish to thank all those who helped us. Without them, we could not have written this book.

First of all, we want to say thank you to the London Meditation Community: the people who have attended our courses, classes and a wide variety of events over a number of years. Because of their feedback, we have developed professionally. It was this that led the publisher to invite us to write this book.

We also want to say thank you to our inspirational teachers over many years: Jon Kabat-Zinn and Saki Santorelli, Florence Meleo-Meyer, Melissa Blacker and Bob Stahl.

And last but not least, Anita Dickinson, for giving our thoughts the right English (native speaker) expression.

About the authors

Albert Tobler has 32 years experience of meditation and is a trained deacon (church officer). He works in learning and development and as an accredited executive coach.

Susann Herrmann trained as a banker and psychologist, as well as in group dynamics. She now leads a wide range of mindfulness training programmes. Together, Albert and Susann co-founded and run the mindfulness-based business London Meditation, "the oasis of light, calmness and inspiration".

www.london-meditation.co.uk

PART ONE

Mindfulness now

1

Mindful living: an introduction

Mindfulness has become a buzzword in Western medicine, psychology, national healthcare services and even in the military. It is increasingly recognized as an effective way to reduce stress, increase self-awareness, enhance emotional intelligence and effectively handle unpleasant thoughts and feelings.

What is mindfulness?

Although mindfulness has only recently been broadly embraced in the West, it is an ancient practice found in a wide range of Eastern philosophies, including Buddhism, Taoism and Hinduism, as well as in Christianity. Mindfulness involves consciously bringing awareness to the here and now, and doing so with an openness, rather than in a "focusing" way.

Jon Kabat-Zinn, a world authority on the use of mindfulness training in the management of clinical problems, describes mindfulness as: "paying attention in a particular way, on purpose, in the present moment – and non-judgemental-ly." We'll come back to what it means to pay attention "non-judgmentally" later on in this chapter.

Mindfulness is about waking up, connecting with ourselves and appreciating the fullness of each moment of life. Kabat-Zinn also describes it as "the art of conscious living". It is a profound way to enhance your psychological and emotional resilience and increase your life satisfaction.

Living in the present

Many of us spend most of our lives focused either on the past or on the future, paying very little attention to what is happening in the present. This means that we may be unaware of much of our experience most of the time. Mindfulness is the practice of staying in the moment, spending more time present to ourselves, and our surroundings. Not trying to change things but trying instead to accept the way that things are.

Mindfulness is for anyone who wants to become more and more aware of themselves, anyone who wishes to improve their health and wellbeing. It has been proven to be useful for people with specific health problems, but it can be accessed by anyone at all to improve their overall quality of life, and their ability to live life to the full.

Put simply, mindfulness is about finding ways to slow down and pay attention to the present moment, which im-proves performance and reduces stress. It's about having the time and space to attend to what's right in front of us, even though many other forces are trying to keep us stuck in the past or inviting us to fantasize or worry about the future. It's about a natural quality each of us possesses, one which we can further develop in just a few minutes a day.

The benefits of mindfulness

Practising mindfulness helps us:

* to be fully present, here and now
* to experience unpleasant thoughts and feelings safely
* to become aware of what we're avoiding
* to become more connected to ourselves, to others and to the world around us
* to increase self-awareness
* to become less disturbed by and less reactive to unpleasant experiences
* to learn the distinction between us and our thoughts
* to have more direct contact with the world, rather than living through our thoughts
* to learn that everything changes; that thoughts and feelings come and go like the weather
* to have more balance, less emotional volatility
* to experience more calm and peacefulness
* to develop self-acceptance and self-compassion

Paying attention "on purpose"

First of all, mindfulness involves paying attention "on purpose". It involves a conscious direction of our awareness. We sometimes talk about "awareness" and "mindfulness" as if they were interchangeable terms, but that's not exactly what they are. So let us be a bit more specific.

We might, for example, be aware that we are irritable, but that wouldn't mean we are "being mindful" of our irritability. In order to be mindful, we have to be purposefully aware of

ourselves, not just vaguely and habitually aware. To
we are eating is not the same as "eating mindfully"

Let's take that example of eating and look at it
er. Eating is something we all do several times a day, something that most of us take for granted. When we're eating
non-mindfully we may in theory be aware of what we're
doing, but we're probably thinking about a hundred and
one different other things at the same time. We may also be
watching TV, talking to somebody or reading a magazine.
Or even all three.

So only a very small part of our awareness is actually
occupied with eating. We may be only dimly aware of the
physical sensations – and even less aware of our thoughts
and emotions. That's why we often eat too much, because
we are unaware that we are already full. Because we're only
dimly aware of our thoughts, they wander in an unrestricted
way. There is no conscious attempt to bring our attention
back to our eating. There is no purposefulness.

But when we are purposefully aware of eating, we are
consciously aware of the *process* of eating. We're deliberately noticing the sensations of the food – the taste, smell, texture of it and our responses to those sensations. We might
sometimes notice the mind starting to wander and when it
does wander we purposefully bring our attention back to the
process of eating.

This purposefulness is a very important part of mindfulness. Having the purpose to stay with an experience – whether that's the act of taking a breath, experiencing a particular
emotion, or something as simple as eating – means that we
are actively shaping the mind.

Paying attention "in the present moment"

Left to itself the mind wanders through all kinds of thoughts. They might be angry, or they might express a craving. They might be depressing; they might concern revenge; or they might be self-pitying. As we indulge in these kinds of thoughts we reinforce those emotions in our hearts and cause ourselves to suffer. Mostly these thoughts are about the past or future.

> *The past no longer exists. The future has not arrived yet.*
> *The only moment we really can experience*
> *– the present moment –*
> *is the one we seem most to avoid.*

So when we are being mindful we are noticing what's going on right now. That doesn't mean we can no longer think about the past or future. But when we do so we do so mindfully – so that we are aware that *right now* we are thinking about the past or future. That's an important distinction.

One key aspect of the practice of mindfulness is meditation, which we will come to in due course. But it's worth mentioning here that when we engage in meditation, we are observing what's arising in the present moment. If, during our meditation, thoughts about the past or future take us away from the present moment, we simply acknowledge that this has happened, and just *come back to the here and now* – by purposefully directing our awareness away from such thoughts and towards our present moment experience.

This is known in mindfulness as the "emergence", a term that Gregory Kramer uses in his excellent book *Insight Dialogue*. We decrease the effect these negative elements have on our lives and we create a space of freedom where calm-

In life and work

The practice of mindfulness enables us to:

* improve focus and concentration
* increase self-awareness
* reduce the impact and influence of stressful thoughts and feelings
* facilitate better relationships
* catch self-defeating behaviours, and substitute more effective ones
* become aware of self-defeating thought processes, and let them go

All of this boils down to three major benefits:

* improved performance
* reduced stress
* greater satisfaction in work and life

ncss and contentment can grow. This is paying attention non-judgementally.

Mindfulness: getting in shape for life

So how do you reach this level of non-judgemental awareness? Well, if you had plans to go on an outdoor adventure, it would be wise to try to optimize your physical performance and endurance before you set out into the wilderness. A good place to get yourself into condition would be a gym.

When you go to the gym, you practice formal procedures (exercises) that alter the fabric of your body in three ways:

* They increase your strength
* They increase your flexibility
* They increase your endurance/stamina

When you do an mindfulness "workout", such as the body scan (see box below), you practice formal procedures (exercises) that alter the fabric of your body in two ways:

* They increase your clarity
* They increase your equanimity

The purpose of going to the gym is not to achieve a temporary feeling of strength and flexibility, one that's only present when you do the exercises and which evaporates afterwards. The idea of going to the gym is to gradually and sustainably increase strength and flexibility, in order to get fit.

The situation with mindfulness training – such as the eight-week programmes we'll explain in Chapter 10 – is similar. The real benefit of mindfulness training is not to achieve a temporary state of clarity and equanimity. The real benefit

The body scan

The body scan is a meditative practice to help us get in touch with our bodily sensations moment by moment. We learn to bring attention to the body, part by part, step by step; we directly observe and acknowledge whatever sensations are present.

Whenever the mind wanders off we just bring our attention back to the body and its sensations – on purpose and non-judgementally. In this way we travel through the whole body, beginning from the toes until we become aware of the body as a whole. For a detailed body scan exercise, see p.68.

of mindfulness training is to gradually increase your clarity and equanimity moment by moment. In other words, the outcome of mindfulness training is not to create certain temporary states in consciousness, but rather to develop a certain sustainable quality in consciousness to last throughout your life.

In order to increase your physical strength and flexibility, what would you need to do? You would need to learn how to perform the exercises properly. You would need to do the exercises with regularity. And you would need to maintain your exercise programme over time.

The same is true of mindfulness training. You have to learn how to do the formal practices (such as the body scan) properly; then practise them with regularity and maintain that practice programme over time. The idea is to develop your personal daily mindfulness practice. Mindfulness training and fitness training are in many respects quite close. However, there are ways in which the two forms of training differ.

Firstly, no matter how intensely, or how long, you maintain a fitness training programme, it is unlikely that the strength and flexibility in your body can increase more than two or three times. On the other hand, the quality of clarity and equanimity in your consciousness can grow without limit. Secondly, no matter how much strength and flexibility you have, old age, sickness and injury will eventually strip them from you. On the other hand, when clarity and equanimity become deeply ingrained into the fabric of your consciousness they are, to a certain extent, immune to the effects of old age, sickness and injury.

To summarize, mindfulness training increases your clarity and equanimity and this in many ways parallels how fitness training increases your strength, flexibility and endurance.

Clarity and equanimity

The meaning of strength, flexibility and endurance is fairly self-evident – as is their relevance to the quality of your life. The meaning of clarity and equanimity on the other hand, and their relevance to your quality of life, may not be obvious at all at this point. So let's discuss what clarity and equanimity mean within the mindfulness community.

Clarity can be thought of as the ability to keep track of all the different components of your sensory experience as they arise, moment by moment. By "components of sensory experience", we mean the basic building blocks of sensory experience such as physical and emotional sensations in your body, mental images, internal conversations and so on. At a deeper level of understanding, clarity is a deep awareness of yourself: a profound knowing of your own nervous system, right down to the level of neurons.

Equanimity can be thought of as an "attitude of gentle matter-of-factness" with regard to your sensory experience. Mindfulness practice trains your nervous system to know itself better and interfere with itself less. At a deeper level of understanding, equanimity becomes a radical non-interference with the sensory flow of your own nervous system.

Here is an example of what we mean by bringing clarity and equanimity to the sensory components of an experience. Let's say that, in the course of that big outdoor adventure mentioned earlier, we decided to climb a mountain to get a breathtaking, panoramic view of the ground. At some point on the climb up, a deep part of you grows so tired, it is ready to surrender. Your original intention was to finish, to stand on the summit.

Objectively, your body is still capable of climbing. But subjectively you want to give up. In this case, what are the

Mindfulness and therapy

Mindfulness training has emerged as a powerful, evidence-based tool for dealing with psychological health problems. It has been clinically proven to aid in the treatment of a wide range of clinical disorders, including chronic pain, anxiety disorders, depression, post-traumatic stress disorder, obsessive compulsive disorder, substance abuse and borderline personality disorder.

specific sensory components responsible for the perception "I give up"? Well, for one thing, there are uncomfortable physical sensations in your body that will go away if you stop. How many distinct manifestations of physical discomfort are there? Let's say there are three:

❶ Sharp muscle pain due to lactic acid build-up (this sensation is centred in your legs)

❷ The sensation of lack of oxygen flow due to shortness of breath (this sensation is centred in your chest)

❸ The sensation of weakness, exhaustion or discomfort due to tiredness (this sensation is distributed over your whole body)

So that's three distinct sensory components right there. Are there any other sensory components involved? Well, there's probably some kind of an internal dialogue going on: you're probably "hearing" what some mindfulness practitioners term auditory thoughts.

You'd be saying to yourself things such as:

✳ "Enough already!"

✳ "I can't do this"

✱ "This really hurts"

✱ "There's still so far to go and it's only going to get worse"

Are there any other sensory components besides these voices in your head? Well, you may have some mental pictures or visual thoughts, a kind of internal projection on your mental screen. Maybe you see pictures of yourself lying down resting or sitting with a drink.

Furthermore, the physical discomfort and the internal dialogue may each set off emotional sensations in your body and those are also uncomfortable. The negative internal talk and physical discomfort may cause your body to be preoccupied with subtle feelings of fear, or impatience, or of self-pity ("poor me").

By way of contrast, the mental pictures you might entertain of yourself at rest may create a pleasant sensation of joy – emotional pleasure. So, in this example, the sensory components that give rise to that voice in your head yelling "I have to quit now" are nine in number:

✱ three distinct sensations of gross physical discomfort in your body

✱ auditory thoughts

✱ visual thoughts

✱ three distinct sensations of subtle emotional discomfort in your body

✱ one sensation of subtle emotional pleasure in your body

Now, suppose that your level of sensory clarity is so high that, without effort, you are able to keep each of those sensory components distinct in your total awareness. Suppose also that your level of equanimity is so high that each of those sensory components arises without any suppression on your part. And then passes without any fixation – like a wave.

In that outcome, you would be able to reach the summit even though that will to quit remains strong and persistent. You would have the freedom to ignore it and stay true to your original intention.

2

Why mindfulness works

Let's start this section of our journey with a short look back at the history of the mindfulness approach and why it has become so evident that it works. You've probably noticed that discussion of mindfulness meditation is much more common than it was just a few years ago. You might have heard about it on television, or read about it in magazines, newspaper articles, blogs or online chat rooms. It has become a movement and travelled around the world. Yes, mindfulness has its roots in Eastern religious traditions, but it has become a secular and scientifically proven approach to mental wellbeing.

A short history of the movement

In the US, it all really started with Jon Kabat-Zinn, a professor of medicine who has been a lifelong meditator. In his post at the University of Massachusetts Medical School in Worcester, an hour's train ride from Boston, he developed the Mindfulness-based Stress Reduction (MBSR) Programme in the course of treating patients referred for intractable and chronic pain. These were patients suffering from medical problems for which there was no cure, with no possibility of surgery. In most of their cases, the only prescription was medication in increasing doses, which itself had debilitating, sometimes life-threatening, side-effects. Their lives were dominated by their pain; many of them were weary of life, feeling their situation was hopeless.

Kabat-Zinn developed an eight-week programme teaching meditative techniques and supporting participants to develop mindfulness. And it worked. So well, in fact, that it attracted more and more referrals until, eventually, the award-winning US journalist Bill Moyers decided there was a story well worth investigating. He arrived with a camera team at the University of Massachusetts Medical School and took part in one of Jon Kabat-Zinn's MBSR eight-week programmes. The footage that he filmed was broadcast as part of the *Healing from Within* series at the beginning of the 1990s. It created a lot of publicity and interest from the general public: it was in many ways the beginning of the mindfulness movement.

At the time, people who practised meditation were considered to be on the fringes of society. In the 1960s and 70s, they were labelled hippies. In the 1980s and 90s, they were generally lumped in with the New Age movement, or described as "esoterics". It's very telling of attitudes of the time that, in the Bill Moyers film, one of the enthusiastic practitioners is filmed saying: "Mindfulness is wonderful, even when it is so un-American!"

The Mindfulness-based Stress Reduction Programme began the process of development of a range of programmes and an acceptance in the wider community of an age-old approach once seen as the preserve of an eccentric few. Today, people who meditate aren't seen as remotely eccentric; if anything they tend to be thought of as progressive and open-minded people. Without over-generalizing, practitioners of mindfulness meditation are often loving, kind, generous, insightful and willing to help others achieve the same rich and fulfilling lives they have.

There is also the fact that, as mindfulness meditation is a practice and not a religion, practitioners don't have to abandon their current spiritual faith in order to avail themselves of its benefits. Furthermore, mindfulness meditation need not just be about spiritual exploration; it is fully **compatible with Western values** and is proving to be extremely effective for all-around personal development. As our journey progresses, we will have a closer look at Kabat-Zinn's ground-breaking training programme.

Though mindfulness meditation has been around for a long time, and its migration to the West has been slow, its popularity has dramatically increased over the last few years. There are several reasons for this. For one thing, there have been significant **changes in the** social and political environment. The end of the Cold War has enabled more communication between Eastern and Western societies. For another, there have been unprecedented advances in communication technology in the last decade or two. The rise of the Internet has made communication much easier between cultures that previously did not interact very much.

Furthermore, prominent figures have been enthusiastically disseminating the practice. Most notably, the Dalai Lama has been active in engaging the West. Interestingly, a great deal of his interaction has been with the scientific community; he is very keen to encourage scientists to conduct research into the practice, and what it actually does for the brain. To this end, he has been convening annual conferences with the Mind And Life Institute, a non-profit organisation comprised of neuro-scientists and biologists (both Buddhist and non-Buddhist). The Dalai Lama's work with Richard Davidson, a leading neuroscientist studying the brain and emotions, has focused upon the study of happiness, compassion and other positive attributes in terms of how they can be enhanced by medita-tion. Their studies have made use of the cutting-edge brain-imaging technologies used in neuroscience.

Science and mindfulness

The Dalai Lama isn't the only person interested in the links between science and mindfulness. Work has been conducted, and papers published, on mindfulness meditation by scientists and researchers from some of the most prominent colleges and universities, such as the University of Massachusetts, Stanford, UCLA, Harvard, the University of Miami in the US, and the Universities in Bangor, Oxford, Exeter, Aberdeen and Freiburg, in Europe – to name just a few.

Many of the latest findings and developments were brought to light at the 10th Annual Scientific Conference on Mindfulness in Boston, Massachusetts, in March 2012. Here are some of the highlights and insights presented at this eye-opening event.

Stress

Cortisol is a hormone produced in the adrenal glands – which rest just above the kidneys in our bodies. Cortisol's primary role is to maintain energy levels and body functions when confronted with emotional or physical stress. Interestingly, re-search has shown that people who practise mindfulness medi-tation have low levels of cortisol. Quite simply, when a person has a more serene outlook on life, they don't experience stress-related disorders.

Blood pressure

Several studies have revealed that meditation leads to lower blood pressure. And by reducing the risk of hypertension (high blood pressure), we can reduce the risk of stroke. In March 2012, the *International Journal of Hypertension* reviewed landmark studies and recent literature concerning the use of meditation for reducing blood pressure in pre-hypertensive and hypertensive individuals. They found that meditation techniques appear to produce small yet meaningful reductions in blood pressure, either as monotherapy or in conjunction with traditional pharmacotherapy. They also concluded that mindfulness-based stress reduction (MBSR) may also produce clinically significant reductions in systolic and diastolic blood pressure.

Heart disease

Another study, published in the *American Heart Journal* in 2009, showed that mindfulness meditation led to significantly reduced symptoms in patients with chronic heart failure. The patients, who had an average age of 61, that received treatment were found to have lower anxiety, depression, improved symptoms and clinical scores when compared to a control group who had not.

Mental health

Mindfulness has become so widely accepted in the mental health community that it's an integral part of the treatment of various psychological disorders such as anxiety, depression, post-traumatic stress disorder (PTSD), borderline personality disorder and more.

Taking a peek at your grey matter

An MRI scanner is a device that can be used to take pictures from deep within the human body. The test person lies within the machine, which has a large, powerful magnet, which produces a magnetic field. This magnetic field causes the atomic nuclei in the body to themselves produce a rotating magnetic field that is detectable by the scanner. And this information is recorded to construct an image of the scanned area of the body.

MRI scanners are particularly useful because they provide good contrast between the different soft tissues of the body: it's that feature that makes them better at imaging the brain, muscles, heart or cancers, compared to other medical imaging techniques. Furthermore, unlike CT scans or traditional X-rays, MRI does not use ionizing radiation.

Findings published by the journal *Psychiatry Research* in an article catchily entitled "Mindfulness practice leads to increases in regional brain gray matter density" were presented. They reported a study investigating brain grey matter concentration both pre- and post-participation in an MBSR programme. Anatomical magnetic resonance (MR) images from sixteen healthy, meditation-naïve participants were obtained before and after they underwent the eight-week programme. The results suggested that participation in MBSR is associated with changes in grey matter concentration in brain regions involved in learning and memory processes, emotion regulation, self-referential processing and perspective taking.

Immune system
Mindfulness-based interventions can also improve the functioning of the immune system; one study showed that it im-

The BBC investigates mindfulness

A BBC TV news report of January 2012 set out to address the theory that meditation can reduce stress, depression and chronic pain. (The footage can now be found on YouTube.)

A test subject took part in eight weeks of daily mindfulness practice of. The object was to see if it had reduced stress, or any of the chronic pain that the test participant suffered from the condition lupus.

We know from previous research that if you do a meditation practice and you are in a lot of pain it is not that the pain goes away, it's that it becomes more manageable. The pain is displaced and can be tolerated. The team from the BBC turned to neuroscience to see if this could be objectively confirmed; a researcher at the Institute of Psychiatry analysed the patient with an MRI scanner.

The scientist asked the test person to let her mind wander normally and then to meditate. The images are open to interpretation, but the scientist confirmed that the results back up the test person's experiences. You could see a contrast in the pictures of the response areas created by pain before meditation and after: meditation effectively calmed down this brain region. In effect, this confirmed that the test person was feeling less pain – or was at least less troubled by the pain. As she said: "I use it all the time and it helps me with my pain [but] there is something very powerful about knowing there is physical objective proof that it is working."

Critics may chip in that, scientifically, two scans don't prove much. But it is part of a growing body of research that suggests mindfulness meditation can help with stress and pain. And, in fact, even self-centredness: when the presenter of the BBC news article tried mindfulness meditation and was then scanned, the images showed a reduction in the frontal parts of his brain that are associated with egocentricity.

proved the performance of the flu vaccine. The study, published in the journal *Annals of Family Medicine*, focused upon 149 people, most of them women, with an average age of 59. Fifty-one of them were assigned to have mindfulness meditation training for eight weeks, while 47 were assigned to do moderate exercise for eight weeks (such as cycling or running), and 51 were not assigned to do anything.

Then, after the eight-week period, the researchers tracked study participants' symptoms during cold and flu season, and also collected nasal wash samples from them. Researchers found that people who practised meditation had 27 total episodes of cold or flu symptoms, lasting a total of 257 days. And the people who exercised had 26 total episodes of cold and flu symptoms, lasting 241 days. But the people who did neither exercise nor meditation had forty total "episodes" of cold or flu symptoms, lasting 453 days.

Another study, conducted at UCLA in 2008, showed that, in a test group of males with HIV, meditation stopped the decline of T-cell production (one of the contributors to the failing immune system that is HIV's result).

Ageing

Research has also shown that the practice even slows the effects of the ageing process. People who meditate tend to look and feel much younger than their actual age. The practice also helps people tap into their creativity. Researchers have found that mindfulness may have an effect on the length of telomeres – the protective caps at the ends of chromosomes – by reducing cognitive stress and stress arousal. Meditation fostering positive states of mind may bring about hormonal changes, which may in turn promote telomere maintenance.

Mindfulness in society

Given that mindfulness has been proven useful in the treatment of so many ailments and diseases, it's little wonder that it is increasingly being used to complement standard medical care. The business world has been quick to recognize its efficacy. Organisations worldwide are beginning to realise that the practice of mindfulness can help dramatically lower their healthcare expenditures. Companies such as Google and McKinsey Consulting are already incorporating the practice into their health and wellness programmes. They are even including it in their leadership training.

One of the delegates at the Boston conference was the US Democrat Tim Ryan – a man with a mission. He explains in his recently published book *A Mindful Nation* how mindfulness can improve one's life.

"Like many who have tasted the benefits of increased focus, decreased stress and a quieter mind, I was motivated to share it with my family and friends", he writes. "Given my work as a United States congressman, I was also motivated to see its benefits shared on a much larger scale. I recognized its potential to help transform core institutions in America – schools, hospitals, the military and social services." He felt that the simple practice of meditation could help his constituents face the many stressful challenges of daily life, such as economic insecurity, the pain and frustration of being unwell, or the responsibilities of taking care of sick relatives in a broken healthcare system. He also believes that mindfulness meditation can have educational benefits: that it can meet the challenges of teaching children to pay attention and be kind to themselves and others in a world full of distraction and aggression.

Mindfulness is revolutionary, but it's not a revolution fuelled by anger. It's a peaceful revolution, being led by ordinary people: teachers in schools; nurses and doctors in hectic emergency rooms, clinics and hospitals; counsellors and social workers in tough neighbourhoods; and corporate, military and political leaders. You might be wondering what is so special about mindfulness, that it can supposedly achieve all these amazing results. Why does this very old concept called mindfulness work at all? What does it do to your brain to produce such seemingly magical effects?

The scientific proof

Zoran Josipovic is a neuroscientist conducting research into the physical effects of meditation upon the brain. When he examined the brains of Buddhist monks with a scanner, it was found that the organisation of their brains looked different to that of non-meditators. Why is that? Because they simply practised attention and awareness a lot by breathing in and out, the response areas of their brains to both internal and external sensations were calmed down. As a result of this practice, your mind becomes much less overactive and is calmer. It is the calm mind that allows sharpness and profoundness of thoughts. Overactivity is a disadvantage for anybody who is expected to make sustainable decisions. It is the cool head that is able to take strong decisions; and tranquillity is the source from which strength rises.

To explain why this is, you need to think of the brain as being composed of three separate areas:

❶ **The intrinsic network**
This is responsible for monitoring inner body functions and it can be trained by practising the body scan. If you

don't train this area, you will experience the symptoms that accompany whatever happens to your body coming and going with whatever intensity they bring. If you train in mindfulness, thoughts, emotions and feelings can be simply accepted and experienced from a distance.

❷ The extrinsic network
This is in charge of what information is coming in from around us. We use it while driving a car, for example. (It would prove fatal not to!)

❸ The default network
This is what we engage when we're not using the first or second but are simply awake. It is the state we are in when we are meditating.

The extrinsic portion of the brain becomes active when individuals are focused on external tasks, like playing sports or pouring a cup of coffee. Research suggests that experienced meditators have the ability to keep both the intrinsic and extrinsic neural networks active at the same time during meditation – that is to say, they have found a way to lift both sides of the seesaw simultaneously. This ability to channel the internal and external networks in the brain concurrently may lead a practitioner to experience a harmonious feeling of oneness with their environment.

3

Conditions for
mindful living

This chapter orientates the reader into a mindful way of thinking. It tells you what you need to be aware of before you commence and gives some expectations of what does – and does not – lie ahead.

Recognize this picture?

In the morning, you decide to do something. In the evening you suddenly realize that you haven't done it. You simply forgot. As a result, you feel frustrated and angry with yourself. It's rare that we are conscious of these little frustrations as we plod on through our lives; we generally function as though we are on automatic pilot. The route is already planned, so we follow our usual patterns. We do not self-regulate; our actions are automatic. In order to live a self-regulated life, we need to give ourselves the ability to make our own decisions. When we react automatically all day long, we do not arrive at a state in which we can make conscious decisions.

Making a map

A good exercise to encourage personal mindfulness is to map out your actions, feelings and thoughts.

❶ Take a piece of paper and separate it into four columns.

❷ Title these columns time, actions, feelings and thoughts.

❸ Set an alarm to remind yourself to note what you feel, what you do and what you think in a particular moment.

It is best to start taking notes every four hours. In the beginning that might mean maybe completing the exercise two or three times a day. Later on you can increase the frequency of your note-taking until your current situation can be noted in a flash.

That way you can improve your mindfulness step by step. It is very important to do this practice in writing. Even if you just try to do it once a day, you will be amazed at how in touch with yourself you can feel by concentrating on your consciousness in this way. We have compiled a map of our own, by way of an example, opposite.

What is missing is mindfulness of ourselves: being able to fully sense and experience our own actions, emotions and thoughts. We need to maintain contact with ourselves; to appreciate what we feel, what we do and what we think. When we are closest to ourselves and able to sense things consciously, then conscious decisions can be made. We can act against the automatic behaviour that is not always good for us.

e	Actions	Feelings	Thoughts
akfast)	Pouring cornflakes and milk into a bowl; grasping a spoon; bringing a spoonful to the mouth; chewing; and swallowing	Hunger; anticipation; sensations of crunchiness, pressure, changing texture; excitement; aftermath of taste	Looks delicious; don't have time, have to get the bus; that bloody meeting; date with X tonight
of after h)	Filling the kettle with water; putting it on; putting the teabag into a cup; waiting for the water to boil; pouring the hot water into the cup; waiting for the tea to steep; disposing of the teabag; pouring the milk; first sip	Anticipation; anger; pressure; relief; boredom; insecurity; relief; smell; taste; warmth; comfort	I need a cup of tea; kettle always empty; where is the bin?; hope there is milk today; that's good!
ing a le of)	Scanning the shelves; spotting the bottle; taking it over to the till; waiting for the cashier; taking the wallet out of the bag; handing over the money; getting the change and putting it back in the wallet; putting the wine in the bag; leaving the shop	Expectation; fear; relief; boredom; anger; relief; rush; guilt; anticipation	No, not sold out? Ah, there it is! I already know the price. Why didn't I say goodbye to the shop assistant?

Finding time

There are no special requirements in order to practise mindfulness. The only thing you need is time and a little silence. "But I don't have any time!" comes the inevitable reply. "And where can I find that silence in my vibrant life?" It's true that we're all increasingly busy; and not many of us are lucky enough to live in tranquil, peaceful environments. But you might like to think about what time you really do have. That "waiting time", for instance: the time we waste waiting for another event to happen. That might be waiting for a meeting to start, or for a bus to arrive; this is time that could be used for an informal mindfulness practice. So there's no excuse of having no spare time to be mindful – okay?

It varies from person to person whether to practise for five minutes, thirty minutes or even more, depending on the time you want to invest. Shorter times are better for beginners because, like most other activities, mindfulness needs practice and time to get used to it. You can do these practices wherever and whenever you like. Once you know how it works, informal mindfulness practice can be done anywhere at any time.

Finding awareness

You begin by not judging things. What matters is to take whatever happens to you in your stride, to adopt the role of a neutral observer – of a witness. Normally, we tend to classify the things that happen to us as either good, bad or indifferent. We try to avoid the bad things and improve the good ones. The indifferent things we barely register at all. This classification happens according to our experience, attitudes and prejudices. So we tend not to question our labelling of these events. Our judgement pre-exists before we have even reflected upon it.

The effort not to judge things, on the other hand, takes us away from familiar attitudes and "educated" thinking processes. By practising mindfulness, we try to give every situation and inner reaction the same attention. This means that we become clear about our own evaluation processes. Of course, taking on the role of a neutral *observer* should not mean taking a neutral *position* on everything.

A mindful person does not tolerate all,
but is able to make decisions on solid ground.
*The **process** of judging things is registered. And when we can*
sense something mostly free from our own prejudices then we are
aware. Mindfulness processes need their time and their rhythm.

Finding patience

We probably all recognize the "Hooray Effect". "Hooray, I've got it!" we want to shout when we have finally understood something or achieved something. One knot is undone. But it must be remembered that such insights come when the time is right and not before. When we are stuck, when we are struggling to find a solution to something, then we must remember to be calm.

This is a very important tool for informal mindful practice during the day. We practise in order to build up patience with ourselves. To be able to sense your own impatience is the key. This observing of one's own impatience is an activity that needs to become very conscious.

You might find you are asking yourself questions about how long a meditative training course ought to take. How long should it take to learn some theory, a few breathing practices and some of the standard techniques, such as motionless sitting and mindful walking? Surely this need not take years?

Well, it may be a fast process to learn some theory but to understand it fully, to take it in and develop it until it becomes an inner posture takes time. To develop an inner attitude from practice takes time. It takes a lifetime. Perhaps the words of the well-known **Serenity Prayer** might help here:

We ask for the grace to accept with serenity
the things that cannot be changed,
the courage to change the things that can be changed,
and the wisdom to distinguish one from the other.

This prayer was published by a minister in the 1950s, and has been part of the Christian oral tradition since much earlier. But it has been adopted by all kinds of secular institutions and incorporated into twelve-step programmes as a sensible mantra and a useful memo to self.

When we keep its message in mind, we are considerably closer to mindfulness. The insight about the importance of patience is not new and is a common thread across cultures and religions in reflections on wisdom. Everything has its time. Do we have the patience to accept that yet?

The "beginner's mind"

This is a completely non-judgemental attitude; one which experiences every impression anew. When a young child sees a flower, he or she explores the flower: seeing, smelling and feeling it as if for the very first time. (After all, it may well *be* the first time they've encountered that particular type of flower.) This attitude makes the world in some way special. It makes mundane, everyday things seem astonishing. The beginner's mind does not assume that things are identical or that near-indistinguishable experiences are repetitious. Irrespective of what the phenomenon might be – a job, a relationship to another person, the hearing of a piece of music for the tenth time, or a meditation experience – the beginner's mind sees things afresh.

Everything is newly experienced. Nothing is repeated. That is *not* to say that we should be constantly going out of our way to seek out novelty; or that routines aren't useful or helpful; or that we should be ignoring everything we know. It would be stupid, after all, to deliberately try to drive your car as though you were a complete beginner. If we had to begin every day completely new to our profession it would be disastrous.

But to make new experiences and be open to them is the target of the beginner's mind. The world simply becomes more exciting. It keeps inviting us to discover something new in every moment of the day.

Opening up to the possibilities of a beginner's mind is an essential part of mindfulness; but it is also perhaps the most difficult part of practice. This may be especially difficult when dealing with other people – and particularly with people we do not get on with at all. Trying to adopt a beginner's mind in dealing with individuals we may not even like can quickly become a frustrating task. So it needs a lot of work.

Finding trust

During your practice of mindfulness, you may find yourself doubting the whole concept. "Can I do this?", you might ask yourself. Often mindfulness may appear to be not working. It is not always as magical as you imagine it to be. Then the questions will mount up – whether this all makes sense, whether meditation practices work and whether you should be doing them at all. These are questions that may be diverse but which cause the same blockages on the way towards a more conscious life. Here, what's important is confidence and trust that the chosen path leads in the right direction; even when there appears to be no progress.

There are a number of techniques that support your way to mindfulness, such as the core mindfulness practice of the body scan (see p.68). These make you familiar with your own body so that familiarity with your own person increases. By practising a lot you can keep approaching yourself. You realize that you are becoming increasingly independent of "external authorities" such as teachers, parents, good friends, idols, role models and the everyday aspects that influenced your world previously.

Practising mindfulness does not mean you become a "**self-help junky**". Instead, it increases your trust in yourself and in your capacity to develop your own inner teacher.

Not clinging on

Not judging, developing your patience, keeping the beginner's mind and learning to trust are all attitudes that can be enhanced through mindfulness. But **not clinging on** is perhaps the hardest aspect of mindfulness to achieve outside of meditation.

The whole point is not to blindly follow a target. If you work towards a target that limits the sensations and possibilities around you, you are not able to see beyond, to the world of possibilities that may be open to you. By attempting to reach a target, you focus solely on one particular way because you are not open to alternatives.

We are probably all programmed to set ourselves targets, to keep these in focus and to remove barriers along the way. The idea of not clinging onto preconceived notions and approaches contradicts our usual ways of thinking completely. That makes practicing it difficult.

When going into a mindfulness meditation practice, you should free yourself from expectations. In the practice, things simply are as they now are. If I feel good, it is as good as when I dont' feel good.

Motivation for living mindfully: get ready

This all sounds like hard work – finding time to practise when free time is so rare and life is so fast-paced. You may ask yourself if you can afford all this effort. Please be assured that a mindful life will offer a real return on your investment – a greatly enhanced quality of life. So what are you waiting for? Do you want to prove to yourself that your life is overwhelming, exhausting, senseless or boring? Or do you want to take charge of your life and start to live the life you always wanted?

Mindfulness:

* allows you to find out what you really want in and from your life
* allows you to see your current reality in the light of the options and opportunities open to you
* facilitates your capacity for self-responsibility

These are the foundations for making sustainable decisions. There might be obstacles as well. Failures, mistakes and false starts are in truth necessary for the learning process in any field of endeavour. We don't live in a perfect world, but challenges and failures make successes and achievements even more valuable.

So what now? Ask yourself if you can afford not to switch – at least for moments in your life – into a mindful mode, to get back in touch with yourself; to re-establish the link with your body and mind, continuous companions on the journey called life. Wouldn't this be great? Are you convinced that you need to be able to do this and curious about how to achieve it? If so, then you will have the impetus, the motivation for the excursion ahead.

It's inevitable that, during meditation, your thoughts might start to take a walk. They start to busy themselves with mental pictures or ideas. That cannot be prevented. For example, this thought might arise: "What shall I cook this evening?" Well, not clinging onto it simply means just recognizing this as a thought and then letting it go again. Try not to let the thought develop into specifics: thinking about what is in the fridge and what you could make with what is in there. If you are able simply to acknowledge the initial thought and then let it go, these thoughts will eventually not even arise in the first place. Try to come back again to the present moment and to experience that.

When we cling onto a target, we try to return our attention to the present. Then our attention – our mindfulness – is entirely in the here and now. You may, perhaps, find that this practice comes relatively easily to you. Equally, you may find practices which others can do readily are more problematic. In this, as in other matters, it is wise to accept your own inner experience instead of fighting or denying it.

Learning acceptance

Acceptance means allowing things to be as you find them. Accept your strengths and weaknesses; they belong to you. Acceptance does not create preconditions. That is what makes acceptance between people who live together into a powerful tool. In a partnership we do not say: "You have to change; then I can relate to you." Instead we see their strengths and weaknesses and accept them for what they are. Acceptance does not put up barriers between you and others. Such acceptance should *extend* to others. We treat ourself with the same attitude as we do other people around us. Acceptance, of course, does not mean passivity or resignation. On the contrary, by fully accepting what each moment offers, you open yourself to experiencing life much more completely and make it more likely that you will be able to respond effectively to any situation that presents itself.

> *Acceptance offers a way to navigate life's ups and downs*
> *– what Zorba the Greek called "the full catastrophe" –*
> *with grace, a sense of humour, and perhaps some understanding*
> *of the big picture, what I like to think of as wisdom.*
> *Jon Kabat-Zinn*

Acceptance has nothing to do with fatalism but rather with having a clear view of what is necessary. Acceptance does not prevent us seeing injustices nor should it suppress the wish for change. But it gives us a clear basis from which we can start. Our minds want to hold onto things; meditation requires letting things be and accepting things just as they are.

Jon Kabat-Zinn says:

"When we observe our own mind grasping and pushing away, we remind ourselves to let go of impulses on purpose, just to see what happens if we do. When we find ourselves judging our experience, we let go of those judging thoughts. We recognize them and we just don't pursue them any further. We let them be, and in doing so we let them go. Similarly when thoughts of the past or future come up, we let go of them. We just watch."

These are exciting tasks – for mindful people, at least. But taken in themselves, these attitudes do not suffice to produce mindfulness as a basic attitude. You can practise these attitudes with meditation. However, it would be fruitless to sit and work on one factor after the other by meditating. This is not to reduce the value of meditation in itself. Meditation helps as a technique in practising mindfulness. But without basic sensitivity, an open spirit, the wish to interact with nature and life in general mindfully that is not going to work. As a result, the basic foundation for mindfulness is the inner attitude. For that everyone has to make a personal decision.

4

Understanding the mind and emotions

Let's use a simple analogy to explain the interaction between mind and emotions. Remember, we are embarking on a journey. We know that this journey goes towards our self and towards a more mindful life. But imagine that this was an actual, physical journey. Imagine it was one we were thinking of taking with a few friends. Imagine we had not yet made up our minds about where we wanted to go...

Thinking and decision making

We would need to decide – and agree – upon which country we were going to visit, taking account of such matters as the length of the trip, the costs involved, how much spending money would be required and any specific concerns about travelling as a tourist. So the apparently simple question of where to go has all sorts of logistical implications.

Just as our travel companions would need to form opinions about our proposals, so does the "emotional referee" inside us determine what it "thinks" of our mind's thoughts. At this juncture, we quite often find that our ingenious plan is simply not accepted, because it contains consequences which for ourselves or other participants are emotionally unacceptable. We tend to make our final decisions about a course of action emotionally; the mind and its rationality on their own do not decide anything. This could well be a big blow for our conscious ego.

After all, the ego is conventionally seen as the originator of our wishes, thoughts, imagination and actions, whenever those actions are self-induced. It is regarded as the initiator of our behaviour. Recent insights about the neuronal basics of behaviour, however, give rise to a totally different picture: rationality and logic may provide the arguments to spur us onto one or other course of action, but they ultimately decide nothing definitively. The more important a decision is for someone, the more they will be led by conscious and – especially – *unconscious* feelings. These feelings are short messages from our emotional "experience recall".

This emotional experience recall might be seen as a type of rationality in itself. Though it's an emotional response, it is, in one sense, not entirely different from ordinary rational thinking – because it is based upon experiences that we have learned from; things that have been proven from an individual's perspective in life until to date. The different experiences that different individuals have had shape their assessment of the behaviour of their fellow human beings – and their own behaviour. Whether that behaviour appears reasonable or not is ultimately coloured by our experience recall.

None of this should be seen as a deprecation of rational thinking – and especially not of logical thinking. Mind and

The limbic system

The limbic system is a network of structures located beneath the cerebral cortex. This system is important because it controls behaviours that are essential to our lives; it is involved in motivation and emotional behaviours.

While the structures in this highly developed part of the brain interconnect, research has shown that the amygdala, a small almond-shaped structure deep inside the brain and the hippocampus, a tiny, seahorse-shaped structure, seem to be the main areas involved with emotions.

The amygdala connects with the hippocampus as well as the medial dorsal nucleus of the thalamus. These connections enable it to play an important role in our coordination and control of major activities related to emotions and to the expression of mood.

rationality are extraordinarily important, preventing us from reacting over-spontaneously and prematurely; allowing us to analyse complex situations thoroughly and to pursue relevant complex action planning. For this reason the advice to "be mindful" is good advice. However, there is no guarantee that the limbic system – that part of the brain which governs emotions – will concur with the processes of the rational mind.

That depends solely on what kind of advantages or disadvantages the limbic system, in the light of previous experiences, hopes to gain from so doing: to what extent these processes are connected with strong positive or with strong negative emotions.

Being or doing: an eternal dilemma

At the heart of all this lies a classic human dilemma: between being and doing. At the level of the ego, we like to express ourselves as creative and active; we like to think of ourselves as people who are shaping and forming our own lives and the environment around us.

All animals other than man simply get on with just existing. But humans are not happy just to be; we have to be always doing something or achieving something. Doing something is not letting it be. Doing is an attempt to change a situation, which may well be appropriate when the situation is an external one.

However, when the situation is internal – that is, a state of being – trying to change this state by *actively doing something* gives rise to internal conflict. If we act upon our self, one part of the personality will invariably turn against another part. Our ego resists, turning against the body by using its will against the sensations of our body. Symptoms of physical illness or psychosomatic disorders may be the consequences. In this way we split our whole being and thereby we are weakened.

Using our will to suppress our feelings may be necessary – when we are facing real danger, for example, in which case it is expedient. We need to overcome our feelings simply in order to survive in those kind of situations. But it becomes unhealthy when we are persistently manoeuvring in this way in our day-to-day life. Many people are engaged in a permanent battle with themselves – engaging their willpower to bring about change but in a way that only serves to deepen the split within themselves. Research has made it evident that emotional health can be gained through self-awareness and self-acceptance; benefits gained through continuous mindfulness practice.

There is a process of change that takes place from within and requires no conscious effort. It is known as **personal growth** and it enhances being instead of splitting it. It is not something we can do actively and it is not therefore a function of the ego *but of the body itself*. Again, we need to remember here that the emphasis lies on "not actively doing". What we can "do" is allow it to happen.

Imagine a little, fragile shoot in a garden. Would you pull it up because you can't wait for it to grow? Or would you rather nourish it and care for it to see it grow in its own time? Well, it is the same with personal growth: we can train our mindful skills such as patience, the ability to witness non-judgementally and our capacity of letting go. And it is exactly the new quality of our awareness that lets us recognize the changes in ourselves and through the responses we get from the people around us.

Therapeutic change is similar to personal growth in that it is an internal process that cannot be accomplished by conscious effort. A therapeutic change in mindfulness has to do with healing from within. Growth in mindfulness (and not only in mindfulness) is an enhancement, a further development. Therapeutic and personal growth may be comparable processes but they start from different preconditions. They also have different intentions: therapeutic approaches are used for relief and growth seeks advancement.

This is not to say that doing plays no role in our personal growth process. For example, in the process of learning a skill it is necessary to perform certain actions consciously, so that our learning can be successful and sustainable, but the learning itself takes place on an unconscious or bodily level – it becomes an unconscious competency.

Our ego works by setting goals and controlling the actions needed to achieve them. If the goals become secondary to the actions, the activity lessens and we are shifting from doing to being. All productive activities such as working in the office or growing organic vegetables are aspects of doing.

But when pleasure is the dominant motivation – as, for example, when we are dancing or listening to music – our activity requires less and less effort and the act transforms from doing to an aspect of being. That happens, for example, when a dancer becomes so connected with the movements that they can almost be said to have become the dance itself. When a marathon runner is "entering the zone", he or she is aware that these legs and these feet are doing the job – but that this spirit is free. These are the moments in which we can catch a glimpse of our goal: fully being in the here and now.

Being equated with feeling

We cannot make or produce a feeling, any more than we can create being. Genuine feelings arise spontaneously (even if what gives rise to them is stimulated artificially). At the same time, feelings do not produce or accomplish anything; there is neither goal nor purpose to feelings. We can give reasons for our feelings, but our feelings do not arise in response to the dictates of reason. They often occur in opposition to reason. They are spontaneous chemical reactions in the brain and bodily sensations responding to the world around us. Their function is to sustain and enhance our life's process.

Our conscious activities, our doings, may actually block or inhibit feelings. Our actions are often dominated by the goals we seek to achieve and feelings are seen as irrelevant. However, we have all had experiences where – particularly in the short term – our feelings have impeded our performance. That explains why people try to transform themselves into emotionless machines until they have achieved their goal in the (mistaken) interests of greater efficiency.

But in the long run, when we continually try to avoid our emotions and feelings it may well lead to a kind of permanent inability to experience these important bodily sensations. The other side of this is that there is also a positive message. Because when we pay at least as much attention to our processes as to our goals, then our action-taking can transform itself into a creative or self-expressive state; one which enables us to increase our sense of being.

In terms of being, what counts is not *what* we are doing, but *how* we are doing it. Our doing may enhance our self, but if we do not have a sense of self, of our own individuality, our doing will not compensate for the lack. We cannot become an authentic person by doing. Our life will prosper in the balance between *making it happen* and *accepting it as it is*. Mindfulness can help us to find a better way of handling our feelings and emotions and to take better care of ourselves. Indeed, how we treat ourselves is an important feature of mindfulness.

Everyday mindfulness

Practising mindfulness in our everyday lives can lead to a significant enrichment of life. In our everyday activities, we can use mindfulness deliberately to get in touch with the current moment. When we are eating, showering or walking we can bring our awareness fully onto what is now taking place; this activity allows a conscious and enriching experience.

Let's take the example of walking. If you spend a few minutes thinking about the way you walk, you can experience this activity in a whole new way. When walking, we can ask ourselves questions such as:

* What is my mobility like? Is it hard or easy? Do I shuffle or spring along? Do I go slow or fast?

* Am I rushed or relaxed? As my feet touch the ground, how do they hit the ground? How do my feet roll as they lift?

✳ How is my posture when walking? Am I straight or crooked? How do I hold my head and arms? Are both shoulders at the same height? Do my arms dangle?

✳ How does it feel to walk? In what kind of mood do I find myself? Is this mood reflected in the way I'm walking? How does it feel to go faster or slower; to hop or run?

To practise mindfulness we must be ever more willing to meet common activities with an increased attention to detail and attention to our own being (and wellbeing). In many ordinary moments, we can stand back – or sit back, or lie back – and allow ourselves to be self-aware; we can ask questions such as:

✳ How am I really right now?

✳ Am I sitting comfortably?

✳ How long have I worked without a break?

✳ Should I just go out and get some fresh air?

If you adopt this approach, it should eventually become habitual. You start to pay attention to taking care of yourself. At once, more choices are available to you; you will be aware and able to make decisions based on your own real needs.

Mindfulness and feelings

At the beginning of our mindfulness training, we need to accept certain things. One is that we have very little control over our emotions. We cannot really influence exactly what occurs when a particular emotion – such as fear, sadness, but also joy – arises or when it will cease. Often we are confronted with a *fait accompli* with regard to our feelings. And when we try to escape or to subdue or to avoid certain feelings, this often leaves us even more miserable, and probably frustrated as well.

A more careful handling of our own feelings would help us to see these feelings for what they are. They are neither right nor wrong; they are just there. They want nothing other than to be perceived. Psychosomatic symptoms often arise precisely from attempts to maintain control over our own feelings. Mindfully observed activities can help us to perceive emotions in everyday life and to identify them in a value-free way; to recognise that there is no feeling or emotion that lasts for ever.

This acceptance of the uncontrollability and transitoriness of feelings and emotions supports us and allows us not to succumb to the illusion that we can actually take control. This approach also helps us not to become overwhelmed by feelings and make decisions that will be regretted later. In the here and now, it allows us to decide freely and consciously select from the options genuinely available to us.

Self-care

Another crucial aspect of mindfulness practice is self-care. This means taking good care of ourselves, giving ourselves attention, recognizing our own needs and respecting them. Central to this is self-acceptance – having a positive attitude towards ourselves. This includes satisfaction with oneself, appreciating our own opinions and reactions and feeling at home in ourselves.

Importantly, self-acceptance is also necessary for our own supposed weaknesses or errors. A basic requirement for this positive regard for oneself and loving contact with our self is mindfulness, our own sense of increased attention and sharpened perception. Through mindfulness we imbue ourselves with positive attention for ourselves – especially for our own feelings and needs. We need to practise showing a loving devotion to ourselves, as we tend to otherwise only do so for others who have a special meaning in our lives.

With regard to your body, you might ask:

* How do I feel about my body?
* How is my body doing right now?
* What do I perceive?

With regard to your feelings and needs, you might ask:

* What do I feel?
* What do I need right now?
* How can I do something good?

Achieving balance

Greater care for yourself will lead to an exploration of the way in which you arrange your life; the emphasis you place on the different components of it and the time and energy you devote to them.

It will make you question:

* How much time do certain aspects of my life absorb?
* What time do I have outside of work to do other things?
* What time is there in my life for me?
* To which aspects of my life do I devote the most energy?
* What are my priorities?
* Are these priorities reflected in the time and energy spent on them?

It is often a lack of balance which gives rise to stress or it may exacerbate stress which has its genesis in other factors. If this is the case, it may be helpful, for example to create such things as priority lists and weekly plans to bring life back consciously into a healthy balance.

Indulgence training

Feasting, pleasure and indulgence play a crucial role in our quality of life. Many people have lost the capacity to wholly experience joy, especially at those times when things are not going well in general and comforting moments of enjoyment would really lift the spirits. Mindfulness can help the senses to open themselves up again to pleasure, because awareness is the prerequisite for enjoyment. In order to benefit from a walk, from eating something or from listening to music you have to learn it again. How this works is illustrated by what has become known as the "raisin exercise".

Exercise: the raisin

Take a raisin in your hand, on your palm – or put it on a plate. Now take a close look at this raisin. Look at it as if you haven't seen something like this before.

Turn it over between your fingers, exploring its texture, examining the highlights where the light shines, the darker hollows and folds. Let your eyes explore every part of it. Smell the object, taking it and holding it beneath your nose and with each in-breath, carefully noticing the smell of it.

Now slowly take the object to your mouth, maybe noticing how your hand and arm know exactly where to put it, perhaps noticing your mouth watering as it comes up. Gently place the raisin in the mouth. Notice how it is "received" without biting it, just exploring the sensations of having it in your mouth.

When you are ready, very consciously take a bite into it and notice the taste that it releases. Slowly chew it and notice the saliva in the mouth, the change in consistency of the object.

Then, when you feel ready to swallow, see if you can first detect the intention to swallow as it comes up, so that even this is experienced consciously before you actually swallow it.

Finally, see if you can follow the sensations of swallowing the raisin, sense it moving down to your stomach and also realise how your body is now feeling after eating one raisin mindfully.

When we encounter a raisin – something that we would otherwise wholly take for granted – in this way, it seems to be something totally new. We may be utterly surprised at how varied this experience can be when approached with a "beginner's mind" – or put another way, when we eat the raisin mindfully.

This is a fabulous example of allowing our attention to be focused on the positive stimuli of the present moment and harnessing a sophisticated use of our senses to allow us to access enjoyment. Try this exercise for yourself. This might be the moment when you become aware that:

* I can find joy
* There is pleasure to be had in small things
* There is a world of experience to be explored
* This is me
* Now is the time to do something good for...

Hopefully you are now prepared for, and have a flavour of what to expect from, the next part – the short course in mindfulness which is the heart of this book.

PART TWO

A short course

5

First steps and preparation

We know that it's not an easy manoeuvre to brake suddenly whilst driving at high speed. We know it's wise to drive sensibly so that we can slow down first and brake in a controlled manner. Living in our fast-paced world, we have to slow down before we can pause long enough to relax.

It's worth reminding ourselves that mindfulness is not relaxation. However, we would recommend starting your mindfulness practice from a more relaxed position. Only a relaxed mind and body allow us to be calm and ready to go on the journey to our self. So let's take a deep breath now and find a posture to start our mindful practice.

A choice of four postures

When we want to embark on that inward journey, to become aware of what is there to be discovered, or to become the witness to our inner world, we can choose to do so using a range of postures.

Sitting

This is the most common posture for practicing mindfulness meditation. A particular version of the seated posture – the lotus position – is also the posture most commonly associated with meditation. You can probably picture the lotus position: people sit cross-legged, with fingers held palms-upwards in a particular and very graceful position.

But it is not an easy posture to adopt or maintain and is certainly not essential. Most of us cannot sit long in this pose. It is far more important that you find a posture that is comfortable and will allow you to minimize the chance that you will be disturbed by unpleasant bodily sensations.

You can sit on the floor, on a mat, on a cushion – whatever seems more appealing to you. Sitting with your knees supported by cushions, so that your leg muscles are in a tension-free position, is one position many find comfortable.

It's strange but true: somehow, being on the floor gives you a more "grounded" feeling that makes it easier to calm the mind. The most common alternative to a cross-legged meditation posture is to kneel, having the weight of the body supported on cushions or a meditation bench.

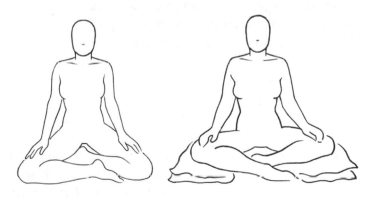

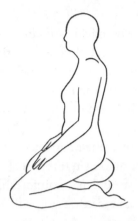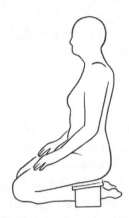

Finding appropriate cushions is important. They need to be really firm, and most pillows and ordinary household cushions just compress too much: they don't give you enough support. However, there are a lot of suppliers (who can easily be found online) that provide yoga and meditation accessories such as meditation cushions, mats and even purpose-made wooden kneeling benches.

Employing the bench is easy. You kneel down and place the bench over your lower legs (i.e. behind you – see illustration above), which are resting on the floor. Then you sit down on the bench. Your legs, and your knees in particular, are now relieved of the burden because most of your weight is resting on the bench (though you are still kneeling).

You can also use the meditation cushions, by kneeling with them between your legs, although cushions can of course be used for sitting cross-legged as well. Most people who choose to sit astride cushions need two or three, depending on the height required.

The important thing is to get the right height. If you sit too low, you'll end up slumping. Slumping interferes with your ability to stay aware and can lead to discomfort. If you sit too rigidly straight, then you will have too much of a hollow in your back, which can lead to pinching. When you feel that your back is relatively upright, but without requiring much effort to keep it that way, then you've got the height about right. Your hands may be resting on your thighs.

You might alternatively use a chair to sit on. It is best if you don't lean against the back but sit upright with a self-supported spine and in a dignified posture. Your feet should be flat on the floor and your legs should form a ninety-degree angle. You may need a cushion under your feet or under your bottom to achieve this, depending on your height (and the height of the chair). Your arms may rest in your lap or on your knees. An additional pillow in the lower back might be helpful to sit straight and upright.

The best way to discover your optimum sitting posture is to try out different possibilities. Feel free to experiment.

Lying down

If you wish to lie down, then lying on a rug or a mat will probably be the most comfortable posture. But it might also be the most difficult for those who are very stressed or exhausted – the danger being that you relax too much and consequently fall asleep. As ever, try it out for yourself; learn from your own experiences.

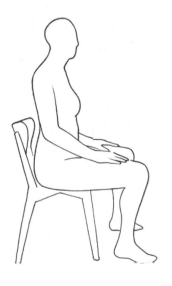

However, when you choose to practise lying down, ensure that you are lying straight on your

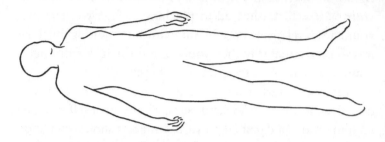

back but not with your feet together, and with your hands along-side and not touching the body.

You may find that lying down like this over a longer period of time is too difficult on your lower back. It might be helpful to try the astronaut posture – so called because it mimics the position of an astronaut when placed in the space capsule for the start of the voyage. In this posture you lie on your back, with your head and back resting on the floor, but with your calves and feet up, resting on the seat of a chair.

If you find that you are getting sleepy whilst in the lying-down posture, you can lift your arms to stay awake. You might choose to lift only your lower arms, leaving the upper arms

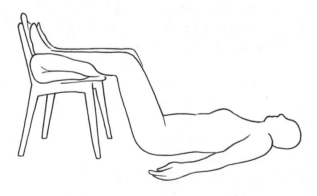

resting on the floor, or lift both arms from the shoulders but without stretching them too much, allowing them to rest on your shoulder blades. When the sleepiness or drowsiness goes away again, release your arms slowly and mindfully and when you become aware that sleepiness is creeping over you once more, raise your arms again.

In general, we don't recommend practising mindfulness lying down on your bed (although it might be quite tempting). Practising mindfulness is about "falling awake" not falling asleep.

Standing

If you want to stand, then stand upright with your arms loose at your side and your shoulders relaxed: that's the recommended stance. Stand with your feet hip-distance apart and parallel, your toes pointing straight forward. Soften the backs of your knees just enough to feel your pelvis relax downward and your weight come onto your feet – as though you had just mounted a horse.

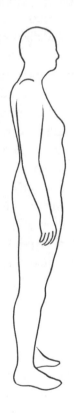

The standing posture is a very powerful posture. Although your mind might tell you that it is too exhausting to stand for a long period of time, you should try it out nevertheless. We can highly recommend it, especially when you want to practise in the evening after a hard day's work. Let's face it, falling asleep in the standing position is far less likely than when you are lying down!

Walking

Walking, particularly in the countryside, on your own and with an open mind, can be very mindful. There is much to become aware of without the need to analyse or even to judge. This is always a great way to indulge your body and mind. However, meditative walking can be done indoors as well as outdoors, because it is a meditative approach on its own.

During meditative walking – which is one kind of mindful movement – we can bring our attention to a lot of different bodily sensations. To keep it simple let us describe here just one option of bringing moment-to-moment awareness to our body while we are walking.

First of all, before you even start moving, become aware that you are standing in an upright posture. Feel your feet on the ground and notice that your feet are bearing the weight of your body. Your hands are loose at your side and the shoulders relaxed. You might notice that your body is shifting ever so slightly to keep its balance.

When you are ready to start, consciously shift the weight of your body to one side, onto one leg, and feel the impact of this shift in your feet – first one foot, then the other. This is just a shift in weight – we're not standing on one leg, or taking an actual step here. One leg might feel lighter, or more "empty" than the other one. Slowly and consciously lift this leg up from the floor and move it forward – in a smooth motion – to place it heel first, softly, on the ground. Let the rest of your foot follow until your full sole is resting again on the floor. Then shift the weight of the body to the other foot and lift the now weight-released leg. Step forward in the same way as you did before.

Stay fully aware with every moment of this ongoing series of movements: shifting the weight, lifting the foot and stepping ahead; and bringing down the foot heel-first in a smooth and steady way. Walk for as long as you like and really dive into this experience. Let the main focus in this practice always be on the sensations in your feet, moment by moment.

You are walking consciously and very slowly. At first, you may find it hard to keep balance, because what your body is used to doing all the time on automatic pilot suddenly takes on a new complexion when it calls for the concentration of your conscious mind. If you want to explore this experience in depth, aim for each single step to take thirty seconds. Absurd? Not possible? Well, it might be a challenge, but it really is worthwhile.

With practice, you will come to the point where you still walk with full awareness but give the control back to your body and are able to relax. This is the moment, when the exercise truly transforms into a mindfulness practice, when we make a transition from walking consciously to observing the movement while it happens.

Additional practicalities

You can practise mindfulness with your eyes open or closed. (Obviously, during a mindfulness walking exercise, we would recommend keeping your eyes open!) We would suggest initially that you close your eyes whenever this feels comfortable, so that you are not disturbed by visual stimuli. However, if you get the feeling you would prefer to have your eyes open it is best that you just lower your eyes and let them rest on the ground just in front of you. But explore what works best for you.

Mindfulness can be practised everywhere – at home, in gorgeous country surroundings or in an urban environment. After all, meditation takes place inside you; it's there that you learn to leave the outer world where it belongs, and that's an important element in developing mindful practice. However, in the beginning, a quiet space is likely to be more supportive and less distracting.

So first of all, seek to make yourself as comfortable as you possibly can, minimizing the chances that you will be interrupted: silence your phone and maybe your door bell, tell your flatmates, if you have any, what you are doing and ask them to respect your privacy for a while. Create your own space!

We recommend, in the initial stages, that you practise at home or in a facilitated group. Once you have had your foundational experiences with being mindful, you will find that you can do mindful practice anywhere: on the tube or bus, on an airplane or train, even at the office.

Sooner or later you will notice that your attitude towards your practice is much more important than your posture or surroundings. If you have an open and honest attitude, if you cultivate a respect and curiosity towards being mindful, your posture will end up mirroring this inner stance.

Formal and informal practice

To be mindful means to face actuality – to be mindful of "what is right now present".This is what we are investigating and observing in detail during our mindfulness practice. We distinguish between two different forms of practice – formal and informal practice – but the same process of present-centred awareness is brought to these two different contexts.

Formal practice involves intentionally stepping aside from your daily activities. It requires setting aside time to practise the skill of simply being with your direct experiences, arising just as they are, moment by moment. This formal practice is the foundation of your mindfulness training.

These direct experiences can include any aspect of our immediate sensory experience, which will include our breathing, other bodily sensations, sounds and the effect of thoughts and emotions on our mind and body. There is no part of internal or external experience that cannot be included in mindful practice.

Our attention can be brought intentionally to very specific, narrow aspects of our experience in order to enable concentration to develop; it can also open out to embrace the broad field of awareness – in any moment.

Informal practice refers to a conscious effort to bring this moment-to-moment, non-judgemental awareness into all aspects of our lives. We can transfer the insights gained in formal practice into practical skills in our daily life. In this context too, we can observe and investigate our breathing, bodily sensations, sounds and other moment-to-moment experiences.

* formal practice is the "laboratory environment". You deepen your experience and "train your skills" of being mindful by mentally observing the breath, emotion, thoughts and bodily sensations

* informal practice is when we can "apply" our skills and insights that we have gained through our formal practice to our daily life (field experience, as it were)

Informal practice can be conducted by really paying attention consciously to our daily routine activities, such as eating, showering, brushing our teeth, emptying the rubbish by walking to the bin and much more.

You will be surprised at how much there is to discover in these small daily routines. Or in the words of Jon Kabat-Zinn: "The little things: they are not so little, they are life!" In Chapter 8 we will continue our exploration of the limitless possibilities of informal practice.

Let's get started

We will start now with the formal practices: they allow us to build trust in practising in general and to gain the skills for the informal practices.

Find yourself a quiet place and make sure you have allowed yourself the time to experience the following exercise step by step: set aside a generous amount of time for it. (You might wish to read the questions in Exercise 1 below, prior to starting the exercise.) During the exercise, try to adopt a mental stance of curiosity and observation. The core of the practice is moment-to-moment awareness.

Exercise 1

In this simple exercise, you will sense your body in its sitting, standing or lying down posture.

Adopt one of the three postures. Pause and slow down, take a breath very consciously and allow your body to settle. Be as motionless as possible. Become aware of how and where your body is continuously moving (breathing, making sounds or, if you're standing up, keeping balance). Now ask yourself:

✳ Whereabouts in your body do you feel is the core of the posture you're in?

✳ How do you know whether you are sitting, standing or lying down?

Try this exercise in all of the different postures mentioned above. Remember:

> *In our practice we only want to be aware.*
> *We do not judge or analyse.*
> *The only purpose is to be the watcher;*
> *there is no other purpose in what we are doing.*

Reflection

When the practice is finished, you may reflect on what kind of insights this looking inside has provided you with. Now you can ask yourself, what does it mean to you? What could you learn from these insights? And how could they be used to bring purpose to your daily life?

It might be that you become more and more aware of, say, your feet on the ground when standing. You might find yourself appreciating this different quality of awareness the next time you are walking. The enhanced quality of awareness is one benefit of the exercise. But this is something to be experienced, not described: description leads to expectations and risks getting in the way of your own discoveries and experiences.

What happens while we are practising?

One common formal practice is to bring awareness to the sensations of the **breath within the body**. The first discovery for many of us is how little of the time our awareness is really in the present moment. The experience of many people in an exercise such as the one just described is that our attention does not remain focused on the breath: it moves restlessly from thoughts about the past to worries about the future; it focuses on discomforts in the body... and so on.

You might wish, right now, to focus simply and repeatedly upon your breathing. We "watch" our breath. And when we find ourselves becoming aware that our attention went off to some other distraction, we consciously bring our attention back to the breath.

Now we are back to "witnessing" our breath. And when, once again, we find ourselves becoming aware that our atten-

What does it mean to be on automatic pilot?

One way to describe it would be by the example of your morning routine. You get up, brush your teeth, shower and get dressed – all without thinking about it. This is good in general, because you wouldn't want to have to consciously think through repetitive and mundane tasks. But the problem occurs when bad habits and behaviours become automatic. For example, if you had developed a habit of waking up each day in a bad mood and thinking negative thoughts, this could have a negative impact on the rest of your day.

A growing body of research suggests that as little as five percent of our behaviours are as a result of conscious decisions. This means that as much as 95 percent of what we do occurs in automatic pilot mode – meaning that most skills and behaviours we learn eventually become automatic habits. For example, when learning to ride a bike, you tried pushing the pedals, but you couldn't stay balanced, so you fell down. If you decided not to give up and practised repeatedly you eventually improved your balance. One day, riding a bicycle became an automatic skill for you – you didn't even have to think about it any more.

This is obviously beneficial when learning new skills and positive habits, but not when applied to negative mindsets and the bad habits we have developed over our lifetime. What if we repeated being impatient with friends and family members, until it became automatic? To break this bad habit, you would need to learn how to get out of automatic pilot mode.

tion went off to some other distraction, we consciously bring our attention back to the breath.

And so on, and so on. This is a simple but extremely powerful exercise. As we do this, direct perception leads us to an understanding of the ways our mind habitually operates. By the process of gently guiding the attention back again and again to direct observation of the breath (or some other aspect of our experience) and bringing an attitude of gentle awareness to all that arises as we do this, we begin to see clearly how states of mind arise and how habitually we relate to them.

This should lead us to the insight into how much difficulty we create for ourselves internally, without even being aware that these processes are happening. We discover how much of our own experience is beyond our awareness.

Much of life can be lived on "automatic pilot" or in "un-awareness" – rather than being awake to the moment. We are lost in our formulations, fantasies, memories, hopes and fears about what is going on, rather than seeing the direct, immediate reality of our experience.

With consistent practice, thoughts, sensations, emotions and all the components that make up our experience become evident. We observe them clearly with awareness and have the opportunity to see that they are events that continually arise and pass away in our consciousness. This simple realization can be very liberating. If we have more of a real sense that everything is always coming and going, we can experience things more lightly and easily. We can also see that it is the way that we relate to these comings and goings that creates many of the difficulties that we are experiencing. We cling to pleasurable experiences or yearn for experiences that we are not having right now; we push away and want to get rid of unpleasant experiences and try to avoid experiences that we do not want; we disengage and tune out in boredom from neutral experiences.

Whenever we react to our experience with attachment, aversion or by spacing out, we will experience difficult emotional consequences such as anger, jealousy, addiction, fear, a sense of worthlessness and so on. All of these reactions and more can arise as we simply give ourselves the space to watch the breath or some other aspect of our moment-by-moment experience. In turn, this gives us the clarity to see how trapped we can be by our own reactions. By enabling us to see our reactivity, the practice of mindfulness creates a space in which we can make conscious choices as to how we can best respond to whatever is arising for us, internally or in the world around us.

The formal practice creates this space more readily for us, by simplifying what we are paying attention to. We are forming our own laboratory in which we can see more easily what is already in the mind–body system. The insights, understanding and connections that arise in this space created by formal practice can then be brought into the more complex world of everyday life.

Mindfulness practice allows us to see that we are more than the content of our thoughts, our past experiences, our bodily sensations, our emotions and so on. All of these things are not who we are! It is remarkable how liberating it feels to be able to see that our thoughts are just thoughts and that they are not "me" or "reality"… the simple act of recognizing thoughts as thoughts – mental events – can free you from the distorted reality they often create and allow for more clear-sightedness and a greater sense of manageability in your life.

This process of not identifying with automatic self-judgements and thoughts leads us to see the "bigger picture" beyond our own limited internal reactions. The awareness is always wider than the content of what arises within it.

The value of cultivating mindfulness is not just a matter of getting more out of sunsets. When unawareness dominates the mind, all of our decisions and actions are affected by it. Unawareness can keep us from being in touch with our body, its signals and messages. This in turn can create many physical problems for us.

In the context of mindfulness, there is a key difference to be noted between mindfulness training and relaxation training. Relaxation is taught as a goal-orientated technique to be used as required to combat stress or anxiety. Mindfulness should not be thought of as a technique but rather as a way of being, which includes all aspects of the individual's life. The practices are taught in ways which emphasize not trying to get anywhere but, for once in our lives, allowing ourselves to be just in the moment, without striving, without actually doing anything – realizing that in some sense each of us is whole and complete as we are.

Mindfulness is cultivated as a way of discovering how to be fully with all of our experiences – pleasant, unpleasant and neutral. Emotional reactivity and the full range of emotional states available to human beings are as much valid domains of meditative experiences as experiences of calmness and relaxation.

The practice of mindfulness for many is undertaken in the hope of arriving at different states, yet mindfulness has no goal but to simply experience what is present, moment to moment. Almost everything we do, we do for a purpose, to get something or somewhere. But in mindfulness this attitude can be a real obstacle. That is because mindfulness is different from all other human activities. Although it takes a lot of work and energy of a certain kind, ultimately mindfulness is a state of non-doing. It has no other goal than for you to be yourself.

Mindfulness is not about changing experience itself, but it gives us the possibility to change our relationship to our inner experiences and thereby enables us to reduce our suffering.

6

The body, breathing and being aware

As we saw at the end of the last chapter, the basic formal mindfulness practice involves becoming aware of the body, the breath, sounds and thoughts. These experiences are always available to us. There is always the body, with its sensations, emotions and feelings. There is always the breath; the sounds we generate and the sounds of the world around us; and our thoughts are present as well.

We continually sense these different experiences, even if we are not aware of them. This is the reason that we work, in our formal mindfulness practice, with the observation of what is present right now in this moment (and, as always, do so non-judgmentally but on purpose).

Awareness of the body as a body

Most of us live mainly "in our heads", and take our bodies for granted (unless we're consciously doing something physical, like working out or playing sport). If the body calls for our attention we try to ignore it. We get rid of bodily sensations that we perceive as unpleasant events, or which we find disturbing.

So it is tremendously important to start by reconnecting with our body to facilitate the heightened awareness called mindfulness. The body is one of our most faithful travel companions throughout our life. If it ceases to function, we are dead. It would be foolish to continuously ignore the advice of a highly experienced travel guide when we are in unknown territory. That's why it is vital that we have good communication with, and understanding of, our body. And the best way to learn its language is to be mindful of its expressions.

So we start by re-acquainting ourselves with our indispensible life support system, the "space suit" that allows us to inhabit planet Earth. The most widely used approach to this, and a key component of formal mindfulness practice, is the body scan.

Different ways to scan the body

The body scan is a very common mindfulness technique. There are different poses or postures in which we can scan the body in a formal practice; we can do it while we are **sitting**, **lying** or **standing**.

Scanning the body allows us to observe the body's own activities and sensations from a perspective of "non-doing", like a watcher – looking from a distance without being directly involved in what is happening. "It's not me, it is the body!" is one way of thinking of it: yes, it is indeed a seemingly paradoxical concept to grasp!

The body scan requires that we become aware of what *is*, while it is occurring in our body and doing so neither analytically nor judgementally; simply observing what arises.

Exercise: the body scan

The body scan is probably the best known meditative mindfulness practice, and develops both concentration and flexibility of attention simultaneously. A full audio version of the body scan is downloadable from: www.roughguides.com/mindfuless. What follows is a slightly shorter version. Here we go:

* This is an invitation to go on an inward journey – to explore the host of your life – your body. This body scan practice helps us to reconnect with our body and to learn how to become more and more present and awake to our physical sensations – whatever they may be

* We invite you just to follow us in this guidance, noticing what is present for you moment by moment, and bringing a gentle acceptance to whatever you may find

* Now choose a position that is comfortable for you. You may choose to lie down on a firm surface or, if you prefer, sit on a chair or even stand. As you do this practice, do so in a state of mind imbued with self-compassion; take care of yourself

* Now sense the breath as it moves in and out of your body, noticing the breath particularly at the abdomen, sensing the rising and falling of each in-breath and out-breath. You might, perhaps, want to place your hands on the abdomen to feel this movement of the breath

* And now, from the abdomen, direct your awareness to both feet, exploring sensations at the toes, in the soles of the feet and the tops of the feet. Noticing perhaps the temperature of the feet, contact between the toes, dryness or moisture, sensations right at the skin and perhaps deep within each foot. And while your body is breathing, notice the sensations in both feet

✳ And now extend this awareness from your feet up both legs, through the ankles and lower legs, the knees and the thighs. You may experience sensations of touch, perhaps an awareness of clothing, of pulsations deep within both legs. Simply notice what is here for you and with this broad focus on both legs, simply breathe in and breathe out. Now move to sensing the tailbone and the buttocks, the base of the lower torso and the pelvic region

✳ What sensations do you experience in this part of the body? Do you sense the breath moving – even here?

✳ Continue moving up the torso from the base to the middle portion of the back and the abdominal region. Here you may be sensing the wave-like motion of the body with each of the breaths moving in and out: the expansion, the returning to the centre at the back and the front of the body

✳ Now, moving further up the body, start sensing the upper back, the shoulders, the entire region of the chest and noticing here what sensations are present

✳ Breath by breath, you may even be able to feel here the pulsation of the heart itself. You may notice the working of the heart in its position between the lungs, the flow of the blood and the freshness of oxygen moment by moment

✳ Moving now from the chest to the shoulders, notice the tops and backs of the shoulders. This is an area where we often experience tension

✳ Bringing your attention down both arms, become aware of the bend of the elbows and the position of the hands. Here you may be sensing contact and touch, temperature – or whatever sensations you are able to feel right here in the hands. Just right here, just right now; hold-

Bodily sensations: unpleasant; pleasant or neutral

When we are practising a body scan (whether full or partial), we feel sensations, and notice whether they are pleasant, unpleasant or neutral. You may have already noticed yourself examining these bodily sensations; the mind often formulates "stories" and concepts around them. You might catch yourself thinking thoughts such as:

* "I feel so relaxed"
* "How lovely"
* "I would like to have this feeling forever"

  or
* "I can't sit anymore"
* "I have to move"
* "Not again, it's so painful"

It is often at this moment that we become distracted by this "mind attack" and delve into one or another of these "stories". Instead, we hold these pleasant or unpleasant sensations in our

ing here, in awareness, the sensations of the fingers and thumbs, the backs of the hands and palms, of both hands and of both arms

* Breathing with this awareness, come now to the region of the neck and the throat. Sense the muscles of the neck, the ability to speak and swallow, to breathe right here at the throat. Perhaps here you can sense your breath at the throat – right at this moment
* From the neck and throat, move on up to the chin, the jaw, the ears, all of the muscles around the ears and the sides

awareness,and simply make a mental note at the back of our minds – a note as to whether the experience is pleasant, unpleasant or neutral (neither pleasant nor unpleasant).

As well as noticing no sensations in specific parts of our body, we might also start to categorize this lack of sensation. At times the mind starts worrying if we aren't feeling sensations (and sees it as an unpleasant experience).

And at other times having no sensations is a relief (a pleasant experience) because we may have previously experienced a lot of pain in our body. At times we experience sensations just as sensations and place them in the category "neutral", because we feel them to be neither pleasant nor unpleasant.

Making such mental notes cuts out the tendency of the mind to seize on potential distractions and elaborate upon them. Once we have made the mental note, we consciously return to perceiving the sensations *as sensations* and progress with our practice. Until, of course, the next "mind attack" hits!

of the head. Continue to the outer ears and the inner ears, being aware of all sensations in all of these areas

❋ Now follow the back of the head to the crown and the entire top of the head, sensing the bones of the skull and perhaps sensing even the brain – the weight of gravity that can be felt right here

❋ Continue the journey to the forehead, the area of the eyes, all of the muscles and skin on the face, the nose, maybe sensing the breath here at the nostrils. Now become aware of the cheeks, the region of the mouth, the lips, the roof sides and back of the mouth, the teeth and gums. You may be aware of the tongue resting on the floor of the mouth before shifting your awareness to sensing the entire face and head – and breathing with this awareness

✳ Now broaden the focus of awareness to include your entire body – from the crown of the head to the soles of the feet, the entire back of the body and the front, the sides, the fingertips and tips of the toes. Fill your body with awareness by breathing in and out as if every pore could breathe

✳ Notice what is present, what sensations are apparent to you. Sense this breathing body and being aware of this experience right here and right now.

✳ Finally, stay with this awareness of your entire body for as long as you want, until you decide that this inward journey, this body scan meditation, is over

Exercise: part body scan

We don't always have the time to execute the full body scan, but it still might be appropriate – from time to time – to get connected with just one part of our body.

When we are worrying or ruminating, when a problem is going round and round in our head, it might be a good idea to connect – even if only for a short moment – with our feet. They are furthest away from the head and allow us to get some distance from the worrying mind and to come back to feeling grounded. And here we go:

✳ Feel the little toes, the big toes and the toes in between

✳ Feel the tops of the feet and the soles, heels and ankles

* If you like, you can expand your awareness from the feet up your legs to include the shin and calf muscles, the knees and thighs

Another time you might wish to carry out a quick partial body scan might be whilst sitting and working at a computer. A lot of this work is done by our hands. So it might be a good idea to place our hands consciously in our awareness for a few moments – and to feel what's going on in all the different parts of them:

* From the little fingers to the thumbs, the palms, the top of your hands, on the surface of your skin and in the bones and muscles

* If you want, you can expand your awareness from your hands up your forearms, elbows and upper arms

After a few moments you can return – with a conscious breath – to your work or daily routine. You will hopefully feel refreshed, reconnected and ready to succeed.

Mindfulness of the breath

There are many breathing techniques around that use **conscious manipulation of the breath** – changing the rhythm and the volume of inhalation and exhalation. In mindfulness we do not alter the breath in any way; we only watch the natural way our body supplies us with air, as the body has done from our first breath as a new-born child and will do until the last breath – whenever that will be.

To be mindful of the breath means simply feeling the breath as it is in the body. From the simple fact that our lungs are working, we can become aware of the related sensations in the body. When we sleep, our body continues to breathe, obviously, even though we are not consciously aware of it. But when we are conscious of our breath we are able to observe it. How often have we really consciously observed the breath as breath?

Particularly when you first start to practise, you may find it surprising to note how difficult it is not to take over, and start "actively" breathing. It is hard for the mind to stay in the background and not be the "doer". But this is what mindfulness is all about – to learn to be and not to do.

Remember that in our observation of the breath (details to follow), we adopt a stance of being non-judgemental, non-analysing – of witnessing. This excercise ought to help us distinguish between knowing on an intellectual level and being "aware".

Exercise: mindfulness of breathing

Awareness of the breath is central to mindfulness practice. We can focus on any area of the breathing process that feels most significant to us. That might be where the air comes in and out of your nostrils, or it might be the way the chest or abdomen rises and falls with each breath. When beginning the mindfulness journey, it can be useful to stay focused on just one aspect of breathing during each practice. The following is an example. (Note: there is an audio version of a mindfulness of breathing exercise downloadable from roughguides.com/mindfulness)

* Sit upright or lie down in a position where you can remain alert and comfortable. Breathe normally and naturally

* Now begin to bring awareness to the breath, wherever you feel it most prominently in your body. It could be at the nostrils, the chest, the abdomen or any other place

* Become aware of the breath coming in and, after a moment, notice the breath coming out. Just be aware of the breath coming in and going out, as it's happening

moment to moment. Simply sustain this awareness of the breath, by breathing in and breathing out

* Now take a few moments to hold this experience of breathing in awareness

* There is no need to visualize, to count or figure out the breath. Just be mindful of this natural process of your body breathing by itself without judgement; simply watch the breath rising and breaking like waves in the sea. There is no place to go, nothing else to do; just being in the here and now and noticing the breath

* From time to time it is natural for the mind to wander from the breath. When you notice this, just acknowledge wherever the mind went and then gently bring your attention back to the breath

* And again now – take a few moments to hold the experience in awareness of breathing

* And breathe, just riding the waves of the breath, moment by moment, and taking this practice one inhalation and one exhalation at a time

* Breathe normally and naturally, without manipulating the breath in any way, just being aware of the breath as it comes and as it goes

* And again now – take a few moments to hold this experience of breathing in awareness

* Decide for yourself how long this meditation practice should last

We also would like to suggest a slightly different variation. You follow the same structure as described above, but this time you decide consciously where you want to observe your breath. You can do it at your:

* nostrils
* chest
* abdomen

From our experience, observing the breathing rhythm at the abdomen is best; this area is the furthest from the head and the region where you are likely to have the deepest experience of breathing.

Mindfulness of sounds

On our planet, silence – the absence of sounds – does not exist. There are always sounds: the sounds of nature, the sounds of our urban or rural environment, the sounds of our living bodies. That's why we use sounds for our formal mindfulness practice, because they are always part of our felt experience, in the same way as our breath is to our body.

In mindfulness, we often refer to the "silence inside". This is a description of the moments when we are able to allow the world around us to be and enter the inner space of calmness and tranquillity: a serene location where nothing exists other than the awareness of being.

Being with sounds as they are

At the start of the practice, consider that your consciousness is like a microphone that picks up everything. You record all sounds around you: laughter, talking, crying, coughing, singing birds or passing cars. You don't think about what it might be good to record and what not; like a microphone, you pick up everything without reservation. The sounds are value-free. For the microphone, all sounds are equal; it makes no distinction. In this practice, simply let the sounds come and go, and notice what happens.

Consciously expand your listening perspective. Become aware of what there is to hear just right now. Hear everything as it is. Open your awareness to all the sounds around you. The important lesson of this practice is that all of these sounds *exist*; they are just there.

It may be that you do not want to hear them; that you experience them as an intrusion in the same way that a fan of classical music may react when someone on the floor above is playing heavy metal. However, you should not consider whether they are pleasant or unpleasant: they are just there. The more time you spend undertaking this practice, the easier it will be just to be with sounds and to accept the sounds around you as they are. You do not have to like them. Just be aware of them; realise that they can be there and that you are not at their mercy.

This practice will strengthen your capacity to cope with life in all its many facets and challenges and to meet what your reality is unconditionally and without prejudice. We will explore this further in Chapter 8.

Exercise: mindfulness of sounds 1

Sounds are mostly out of our control. For that reason, they are good subjects to learn to be with: things that we are unlikely to be able to influence or alter; things that we can only experience.

Let the sounds come to you, don't search for them. Simply notice them, receive them. You may do this exercise wherever you want and you can sit, stand or lie down. It is only important that you find a comfortable and undisturbed position. If you like, close your eyes and allow yourself to "check-in" first. You can practise this exercise for a few moments only or for a couple of minutes. What's important is not how long you are doing it; what's important is the fact that you are open and free of any pressure when you go for it.

In this exercise you are invited to practice:

* Being aware of the sounds as sounds
* Not labelling, not naming, not judging
* Noticing when sounds are arising
* Noticing the presence of the sound
* Noticing when sounds are receding
* Noticing the constant change in the sounds you are hearing

This means that you exercise pure awareness. The idea is to become free of any cognitive/intellectual "doing" and transfer yourself into a state of pure awareness. Labelling – as well as naming or judging – would be a thought process. Remember – here we are experiencing the nature of being, not purpose or reason-for-doing! Keep this in mind before you start this exercise.

Here is an example of how this exercise might proceed in practice:

* You hear a phone ringing on another desk
* You become aware of the sound
* Now a thought arises: "My neighbour's phone is ringing"
* Recognize that this is a thought and not a sound
* You have named the source of the sound – the phone
* Recognize the fact and go back to the sound itself
* Another thought is arising: "It might be an important call!"
* Now you are judging

* Recognize that fact and consciously go back to the sound as sound

* "What a disturbance!"

* Another thought... and another opportunity to bring your awareness back to the sound as sound

Exercise: mindfulness of sounds 2

Here, we will expand our awareness of sounds by using the same steps as in the first exercise, but this time you are invited to experience:

* the sounds *you yourself are making*. Sounds such as breathing, swallowing and slight movements

* sounds in the room you are in just right now

* sounds from outside

Note: these exercises are ideas, tips and hints for how to focus differently and therefore become aware of the manifold varieties of sensory experiences. The main focus of these exercises is the different aspects of the sounds to which we are directing our awareness: aspects such as the sounds as sounds *or* our reactions *or* where they are coming from. And it is in the same way important to *differentiate* clearly, without falling into the analysing trap. We are practising open awareness not comparison, definition or judgement.

Noticing the impact sounds have on you

Sound is a form of energy that is transmitted by pressure variations which the human ear can detect. When a musician plays a musical instrument, say a guitar, the vibrating chords set air particles into vibration and generate pressure waves in the air. If we are nearby we may then hear the sound of the guitar when the pressure waves are perceived

79

by the ear. Sounds can also travel through other media, such as water or steel.

We tend to use the word "noise" to refer to an unwanted sound. The sound of a violin played by a well-practised violinist is considered musical – something pleasing. But the sound of a violin played by someone who is a beginner is often described as being like hearing fingernails scraped down a blackboard. Depending on other factors, sounds may be perceived as noise; noise perception is subjective. Factors such as the magnitude, characteristics, duration and time of occurrence of a sound will affect our subjective impression of it. Noise is a *judged* sound.

Sounds are always around us. If we move inwardly – maybe by closing our eyes and allowing ourselves to listen consciously – we suddenly become very aware of the ticking of the clock, the coughing of the person in the next room, the baby in the other flat, the ignition problems of the car in front of the window and so on.

As we become more and more able to listen truly, we become more and more aware of what really is going on. The result is a clearer and more true reality, with fewer assumptions. If we know we can deeply trust our awareness, we become more self-conscious in a positive and forward-thinking way.

Exercise: mindfulness of sounds 3

In this exercise, the following questions will prompt you to become aware, once again, of how you relate to and react to sounds. You can try this initially during a formal sitting meditation or, later on, when you feel comfortable doing so, in everyday situations.

* Are you aware of the sounds penetrating your ears?
* Do you respond emotionally to those sounds?
* Do you categorize the sound and assess it as pleasant, unpleasant or neutral?

* Do you feel physical reactions to the sound?
* Do you feel a tightening in the face or body?
* Do you feel strained?
* Would you like the sound to end as soon as possible or, conversely, would you prefer it to continue?
* Does the sound generate images in your mind?
* Do you try to find the source of the sound?
* Are you making any judgements about its quality, such as: "What an awful noise!" or "Birdsong is wonderful!"?

Remember: mindfulness is about not judging, but judging will happen again and again while we are practising. So it is important that we become aware of this reaction of our mind – and also that we do not judge our mind in turn for doing it.

Instead, we are simply noticing this natural occurrence and then bringing our attention back to the sound *as a sound*. There is also a audio version of a mindfulness of sounds exercise downloadable from: www.roughguides.com/mindfulness.

Mindfulness of thoughts

Thoughts are the most difficult phenomenon to "observe" in mindfulness practice because it is so easy to get carried away with the stream of our thoughts – the stories the mind is always happily creating. Becoming aware of a thought is the moment when you discover that there is a thought in you mind. Observing a thought means to hold the thought in awareness while it is present in our mind.

We can stay with a thought and hold it in awareness, but this is not an activity so much as a moment-by-moment experience. We can develop our capacity to hold thoughts in awareness purely:

* without identifying with the thought "I'm thinking", or "my thought"
* without labelling (or naming) the thought: this is a thought, after all!
* without judging ("I do not like this thought!")
* without becoming distracted by "stories", such as: "what the hell am I doing here? I have so much to do!"; or "when is this exercise over? Mustn't forget the shopping afterwards..."

This ability increases through practising; we will be better enabled to stay with our thoughts without being interrupted. It's a facility that allows us to become really aware of certain patterns in our thinking, in which we would otherwise be stuck. Once aware, we are able to choose whether we want to live with our thoughts or to change them for the better.

For this reason, it is very helpful to use those elements of formal practice that we have already explored – bodily sensations, the breath or sounds – at various different moments of our formal practice of being mindful of thoughts. Choose one of those three elements to help you at different stages.

Before you start observing your thoughts

You can anchor yourself, using awareness of the body, breathing or sounds on purpose in order to be grounded. It is a good way to ease the transition into becoming aware of the creations of your mind – your thoughts.

During observation of your thoughts

If you become lost in the stories of the mind, observing your body, breathing or sounds, the way we did in previous exercises, can help you to come out of the story again.

At the end of observing your thoughts

Switching your awareness away from your thoughts, back onto your body, or your breathing, or the sounds around you, is a good way to finish this particular practice.

Exercise: mindfulness of thoughts

Simply notice any activities arising in your mind – thoughts in the forms of memories, pictures or daydreams; observe without judging this procession going through your mind.

* There is nothing you need to do with these thoughts, except bring your attention to them; "watch" them

* If emotions or physical sensations arise, acknowledge them and let them be, bringing your attention gently back to witnessing the mental flow

* Think of this mental flow as being like clouds in the sky; your thoughts just pass across your mind. Notice how awareness holds a mental impression – then let it go

When we develop an increased awareness of the body, breathing and sounds, we gain the capacity to have an incredibly positive impact on our lives. Developing an awareness of our thoughts can have an even greater impact. We learn to relate differently to our mental events by challenging them with our mindfulness practice. We will then start to find amazing changes in how we are meeting the moment.

What do we mean by "meeting the moment"? Well, we're talking about the moment when we become aware that we are currently in automatic pilot mode – those moments when we are functioning without thinking, and perhaps not even aware of what we are doing just right now.

There is also an audio version of mindfulness of thoughts downloadable at www.roughguides.com/mindfulness.

Automatic pilot

Remember: our automatic pilot is vitally important when we are driving a car and have to brake all of a sudden for whatever reason. There are a million instances in our lives in which a reaction without thinking is important to survive; when we need to think faster than the time a series of thoughts would take, in order to make an appropriate decision. But when we are meeting the moment, we consciously and on purpose (but without purpose) switch into the direct and open awareness mode. We become mindful; we use the newly developed art of consciously holding our awareness non-judgementally in the here and now.

For example: when a book is being edited and proofread, an author receives comments about how some sentences are phrased, or how a concept is being explained, from the book's editor and proofreader. This book was no exception. Our first response to some of these questions was "why does he not understand what we're writing?" The moment we became aware of our angry feelings, which had evidently triggered this thought, there were two clear options:

❶ The automatic pilot version

To go into the story of "our nagging editor, being pedantic" and spiralling up the negative emotions and consequent negative thought chain.

❷ The mindful way

To pause and watch consciously what's going on within ourselves: an emotion, a thought, body sensations in the stomach and in our heads. By allowing these occurrences to be instead of doing something actively or mindlessly, We become aware of what's really happening. Which in turn brings us back to a calmer state, in which we can make a conscious decision...

And all of a sudden there is another thought: if the editor does not understand a point, many of the readers of this book will also not understand. Therefore it is good to re-think our writing.

The monkey mind

The normal condition in our lives is a lack of awareness in relation to the thoughts we have. The standard state in the Western world is to be deep in thought. While we eat, we might be thinking about having to pick the kids up from school. While we are picking up the children, we are thinking about the forthcoming meeting with our friends, and when we meet our friends, we are perhaps thinking about the imminent and unpleasant appointment with our dentist, due the next day. The crux is: we are never where we really are. We are moving from the past into the future, and the present moment – which is the only moment we can really live in – is the one we regularly miss. The phenomenon responsible for all of this busy leaping to and fro is termed the "monkey mind".

Eastern civilization has an ancient tradition of contemplation – the art of looking inward. The term "monkey mind" (or "mind monkey") is found in Buddhism, and means "unsettled". That's because our mind has the habit of jumping about like a young, impetuous monkey. Within the space of a few seconds, you might be remembering past events, striving to predict the future, and comparing those predictions with what you have already achieved to date. Even just watching these fast mental activities, we can become a little bit dizzy.

Such behaviour is very unproductive and often stress-inducing on the one hand, and on the other hand acts as a hugely powerful filter between you and reality. It is therefore very important to treat all thoughts with greater awareness and to curb this monkey mind.

There is a wide variety of techniques that enable us to challenge this monkey mind, but the essence of most of these techniques involves pure observation of the mind – in exactly the same way that we have previously practised with the body, breathing and sounds.

Thoughts are simply mental events. But we imbue them with power because we see them as telling us truths, predicting the future and describing the reality of our past. If you are beginning to bring your attention more and more towards thoughts, you will gradually come to the realization that these thoughts do not need to have any power over you. With continuous mindfulness practice, their power will diminish and diminish, and your insights will increase.

These insights are manifold: whatever comes up from the unconscious, the place where so much is hidden, stored and buried. Once they are freed and brought into daylight, we can begin to understand what drives us from deep down, day by day, moment to moment.

As long the door is closed we do not know what's behind, and all ruminating, analysis and assamption will not bring clarity – only more abstract concepts of reality. The moment when we pause and bring our awareness from outside consciously inside, we can open the door and look inside – this is what we call in-sight.

One more illustration. If a pond is troubled for whatever reason, the surface of the water becomes non-transparent. The light reflections, the ripples and the stirred-up mud clouds the view. If we are living always with a troubled mind, we never see to the bottom, but if we are able to calm the water, after a while it will be clear and transparent again and we can become aware of what's hidden underneath.

This is why we practise to calm the mind, to become mindful and to become able to see what's really in us.

Stay curious

> *I have no special talents. I am only passionately curious.*
> *Albert Einstein*

Be curious about what you are exploring, however big or small it may appear to you. Curiosity is the engine of growth. We can't find our passions or purpose in life without trial and error experimentation. Curiosity is a mechanism that helps us to create and discover meaning in our life. And in the process of all this we catch glimpses of happiness as it ebbs and flows over the course of our lifetime.

In the beginning, you may find that thought processes are continuously happening, that you "had to" think again and again. Later on, you will be able to let them go more readily. Perhaps for the first time since your childhood, you will become aware again of the world just as it actually is, instead of making assumptions or interpreting what you perceive based on your experiences from the past. It is a long way to go, and takes a lot of practice, but as long as we are "on the way" we will benefit from a constantly growing awareness through our practice.

Through continuing practice – with sensitivity, patience and persistence – you will gradually increase your ability to pay attention. By "attention", we mean those periods when you are inwardly still and simply *present*. You will become more peaceful and joyful and learn to know yourself and your life a little better each day.

Enhancing your formal practice

The important thing is that you make a firm decision – about if and how you will proceed – after either three days or the full seven days without any adjustments. The commitment for three or seven days is fixed.

Daily practice for 21 days in a row will make a huge difference – a difference you will really appreciate. The most important thing is continuity: that this *daily* practice continues over a longer period of time. Really, the duration of your practice is of secondary importance to it becoming a daily exercise: practising for five minutes each day in one week is more effective then practising for sixty minutes once a week. This sustained practice, these long-term experiences, will provide you with insights on a much deeper level and will give rise to a variety of surprising and positive effects on your daily life.

The insights revealed through formal practice

It is one thing to understand, intellectually, the idea of oneself being pure consciousness. But it is quite another thing to recognize this personally and, consequently, to live this understanding. Only when our consciousness of the wholeness and interconnectedness of our being encompasses our brain and nervous system, only when it extends to the last cell in our body, when we have truly realized that the notion of a mind/body duality is not accurate, will we really experience complete freedom.

In order to appreciate this, let us go on a special "sightseeing tour" and explore our body as a holistic organism – holistic in the sense of everything being interconnected. Everything begins when we gently shift our attention from the content of our experience – thoughts, feelings and sensations of the

Your formal practice routine

In our experience, it is very helpful to use the following practice sequence to enhance your personal practice, increasing both its effectiveness and sustainability.

A First of all, decide the object you want to observe in order to strengthen your inner mental muscle. Do you want to bring your attention to the body sensations, breathing, sounds or thoughts?

Then make a conscious decision about the amount of time you are happy to set aside for this practice for the next three days each day.

Once you have decided, don't change or adjust anything. Don't change the object. Don't change the length of time. Just stick to the course of practice you have decided on.

B After having done this practice each day for three days, ask yourself:

Do I want to continue with this specific object?

Do I want to continue with the same length of time?

If your answer is yes, continue with your practice each day for another four days so that you practice for a total of seven days (go ahead to **C**). If your decision is that you want to change something – the object and/or the length of time – you need to make a new commitment of three days (starting with programme **A** again and then progressing to **B**).

C Now you have done the formal practice for seven days without any changes, you can make a decision to go on for an additional two weeks so that you finally have a sequence of 21 days in a row. If, alternatively, you decide to alter anything at this stage, please go back to **A** and start again from the beginning.

body – to *what it is that is aware of that content*. This fundamental shift in attention is what we call self-recognition. We *are* the consciousness which is there before, during and after each experience. We are what identifies any experience as such, but has no experience itself: consciousness.

Remember our various exercises. How do you feel when you turn your attention to the various elements in formal practice such as the body, the breath, sounds and so on? Do you feel lighter and more relaxed? With any luck, you did. It is in these moments that you can observe who is really there when you think of "you". It is the body which experiences; all life is an experience of the body. Thus we can say that a moment in time is an embodied experience. Science tells us that we have roughly 80 billion cells, which are organized in such a way that learning is possible throughout the organism as a whole – it is not only a function of the brain. Learning happens as a process of physical, or somatic, multi-sensory perception. We could turn things around a little and express it this way instead: the body and the entire nervous system is the experience.

The really interesting thing is that we believe that we are the one who experiences things. But mindfulness practices can help us to see that the idea of a "self" is unnecessary – and even inaccurate. When we are relaxed, this habitual focus relaxes, or expands. This sense of "I" is one we can imagine as an interface, which negotiates moment by moment between direct experience and the brain. It enables us to have a temporary orientation, as well as an identity and security. It's actually a rudimentary, natural survival mechanism that is only necessary as long as we know of nothing else.

But this "I-experience" is, in reality, just something we become accustomed to unconsciously. Because of the way our minds work, we tend to narrow our focus and separate ourselves from the object in question in order to recognize and understand the world around us. This habit of tight focusing does indeed produce a feeling of "I". Without this focus, there can be no "I" that experiences itself as separate from other objects. The narrower the focus of our attention is, the more elements of our total experience we exclude automatically and instantaneously. In this state, we cannot perceive many things; we are actually not even aware of their existence. So the narrower our focus, the more we are unconsciously split from ourselves. All that we exclude, we perceive as *separate* from us. We see ourselves as apart, our perception becomes fractured and it appears that there is a mind/body split.

So how does this affect our experience of the here and now? When we are living with a narrow focus, then the experience itself narrows and we feel tight, tense, uncomfortable and isolated in the body. The body follows the focus of attention as a child follows its parents. The moment we relax this focus and allow it to be wide and comprehensive, our experience inevitably is widened and relaxed. The body lets go and becomes soft and permeable. We feel and perceive more and we experience that "being-in-the-body" consciousness much more deeply than we would otherwise.

Most of us have forgotten – or never learned in the first place – what it means to be easily and naturally in our body. Unfortunately, many spiritual paths and Western philosophical traditions downplay, or even reject outright, the interconnectedness of the body. In our experience, the importance of this is greatly underestimated. What exactly does this mean for us?

Many of us do not feel very much at all. We may occasionally experience emotions that can be generated readily by a range of stimuli. But more often than not, our body feels numb; the nervous system has lost its ability to be fully alive.

We opt for a variety of ways to stimulate ourselves, but whatever we opt to do, the effect – seen from the perspective of the connection between body and consciousness – is the same. The outcome of this is a reduced quality of life: vitality only appears as a product of an action, an effort of will, employed to bring it about. We must do something – and we only come alive as long as we do. This becomes a vicious circle.

Somehow we are unconsciously caught in a loop. Everything remains as it was. It is overwritten by activity; by doing rather than being. This knowledge can sometimes be shocking. If we have sought and gained sufficient maturity, we reach a point where it becomes possible to be aware of these somatic levels of experience. And then we have a chance to incorporate the entire body, including especially the nervous system and the functioning of the brain, in the broad focus of our attention. Only then can we effectively integrate all that we still unconsciously exclude – and ultimately gain tranquility. Mindfulness is the way and the decision to follow it is ours.

We need to seek a transformative understanding of the role of the nervous system *in its natural and neutral state*: a state of calmness. Only then can we have a somatic experience of complete freedom. Then self-recognition becomes an experience of more than just a free consciousness; it is truly *embodied*. At this point, the system opens itself to the natural wholeness of life. The separation between so-called intellectual consciousness and so-called worldly consciousness ends. There is a direct, natural and effortless all-inclusive oneness. The whole body, each and every cell, is imbued with consciousness; and we resonate with other beings – with everything that exists. Empathy becomes a natural consequence of being, we are able to mirror our counterpart, and a desire to protect the planet becomes an extension of protecting ourselves.

Then it is possible for us to develop the ability and capacity to deal with everything as it actually is. It lays the basis for true leadership and sustainable development, two topics we will explore further in chapters 11 and 12.

We do not need crutches, concepts, philosophies, techniques and methods any more, to keep us safe and to feel alive. Mindfulness allows us to stand on our own two feet – but connected to what we experience ourselves, to what we see and recognize as true. The quality of our consciousness improves, and we experience a vivid, deeply humane reality.

In the beginning you are dancing, than you become the dancer
but finally you become the dance itself.
Alexis Zorbas (Anthony Quinn), Zorba the Greek *(1964)*

7

The war within

Every experienced mindfulness practitioner knows about "the war within". Beginners will face enemy combatants in this war from the very first moment: difficulties, doubts, irritations, frustrations and distractions whilst trying to engage with mindfulness practice.

After a frantic day, we are totally exhausted and the only thing we want to do is to go to bed and have a good night's sleep. But instead of falling asleep immediately, our thoughts race through our head: scraps of memories of the day, worries, doubts about whether we have done everything right, or fears about what might happen tomorrow. Around one in four adults suffer from **nocturnal rumination** – not being able to sleep due to worrying. Sleep disorder must be one of the most prevalent of the endemic diseases of the twenty-first century.

More and more of us find it difficult to switch off. We cannot quieten the mind. A thousand thoughts fly through our heads. And not only when we are tucked up in bed, but in situations when we really need to keep our cool, such us when we have to solve a serious problem in our private or business life. Our holidays, our long-weekends, our expensive spa weekends are what we pin our hopes to for allowing us some peace. But we may well find that, even during a supposedly relaxing massage or sauna, we're plagued with thoughts of the office, or of memories of family squabbles. When we are hoping our minds might actually take a break – on the couch in the evening, while watching a sunset or when we are taking a stroll in a nearby park – we may no longer be able to find the tranquillity we seek.

Rumination: it's not just the cows...

It is worth remembering that rumination is also the word used to describe cows chewing the cud. Mark Williams, a professor of clinical psychology and a renowned researcher in depression, put it this way: if we drive around the same block for the third time looking for an address, then we are probably lost; if you are thinking about the same problem for the third time, you are probably ruminating. We may believe ourselves to be very close to the "solution", but more thinking will almost certainly fail to get us any nearer to our destination.

So rumination can be described as persistent thinking about the same questions again and again. Questions such as:

✱ How could I forget that I have to pay that bill?
✱ Why did I not put a reminder on the fridge?
✱ What am I doing now?
✱ What if this happens again?

One of the reasons many psychologists and cultural commentators propose for this restlessness is the increasing acceleration of the pace of life of our world; more and more stimuli are to be processed in less time. But, despite our plethora of iPads, laptops and mobile phone apps, stimulation overload is not a new phenomenon; 2500 years ago the Buddha addressed the issue of the troubled mind:

> *The secret of health for both mind and body is not to mourn for the past, not to worry about the future, not to anticipate the future, but to live in the present moment wisely and earnestly*
> **Buddha** *(563–483 BC)*

More recently, researchers and therapists focused their attention on the actual content of our thoughts – as opposed to the factors causing those thoughts in the first place – supposing that it is this element which needs to change. As a result, concepts such as positive thinking and cognitive restructuring boomed. But numerous studies have now shown that these alone may not address underlying problems.

In one recent study, a test group of people were asked to repeat the following positive statement again and again: "I am a loveable person". You might imagine this to be the perfect example of a phrase that encapsulates positive thinking: a phrase that, reinforced by repetition, would leave you feeling more confident, more likely to actually believe it. But the researchers found that after the exercise, particularly insecure people among the group reported themselves to be feeling even less loveable. The phrase they had repeated was ultimately very different to the thoughts within their minds. Thoughts that might be summarized thus: "Actually, that's not right at all; I only have to think about how I was seen just the other day for instance..."

Rumination can, of course, be a healthy activity in life, preventing us from being reckless, or motivating us to do our best to take control of a situation. But some people ruminate a lot more than others, to the point where it turns into plain and simple **worrying**. So what is worrying? Well, we all know the literal answer to that: it is when we turn thoughts over and over in the mind, moodily and at length. It is when we fret about our jobs; mope about our discomforts; or stew over unpaid bills. It means spending a lot of time thinking about bad things and being preoccupied with negative possibilities. The more we do this, the greater our worries become. We may even find ourselves worrying about all the time we've spent worrying!

Worries are basically fears

Everyone gets scared, but we all handle fear in different ways. Sometimes it's easier to dwell on something we fear than to do something about it, or to accept that there is nothing that *can* be done about it. Lack of confidence could be to blame. We may not believe that we are capable of taking action or handling a bad situation.

Our body also reacts chemically to the fear that worrying can create. When we are scared, our body releases adrenalin. This is a result of the "fight or flight" reflex: a vital instinct that we humans evolved over time to help us to overcome or run away from anything that threatened us physically. Amongst other things, adrenalin affects the digestive system and can make us feel ill. The more we worry, the worse it gets and a sudden rush of adrenalin can lead to butterflies in the stomach, a headache or feeling very sick.

Confusion, fusion and defusion

When we feel confused, we are experiencing a lack of clarity; we are losing orientation or navigation in our day-to-day life;

and we may feel anxious, helpless and desperate. Only a few of us are able to deal with this confusion in life – people who don't live by their mind alone, but also from a place of **silent presence**; a place we hope we are making accessible to you in our mindfulness journey.

The mind is an amazing, complex organ, capable of incredible feats of reasoning and calculation. But for much of our daily lives, it is simply a bundle of conditioned responses: its working consists of interpretation of stored-up data from the past. Of course, how we interpret things is very individualistic, depending on our past experiences: there is no objective "ultimate truth" that any one person's brain might apprehend. All perspectives are, in the end, just one of the many perspectives possible for a given situation – no perspective is entirely accurate or truthful.

When we live by our mind, we live in the world of perceptions, and all perceptions are ultimately assumptions of one kind or another. We can try to predict, but no prediction is ever going to define reality. Life is ultimately uncertain. But the mind always seeks certainty; hence the conflict and confusion we find ourselves in.

We need to be aware that there is no such thing as the "right" decision; it is just one of the possible directions that our life heads in. All directions ultimately merge into a path of learning. If our learning is based on clarity, our decisions will become clear and authentic. This does not mean that they will always be "right" in the eyes of others, but at least they will be clear to *us*. Clarity comes through becoming aware and being aware: that is the consequence of living mindfully.

Increasingly, therapists and counsellors are recognizing that the focus should not be on teaching their clients to change the *content* of their thoughts, but on teaching them to win a virtual inner distance from their own thoughts – holding these thoughts in awareness rather than identifying with them. In what have become known as "Mindfulness-Based Approaches" (see Part 4), clients learn to recognize their thoughts as nothing more, nothing less, than just thoughts. "Thoughts are not facts" has become the aphorism.

A thought such as "I could have been friendlier to my colleagues" is not a description of reality, just because we thought it. But usually we believe our own thoughts. Experts call this **cognitive fusion** – we have merged with our thought. If the thought "I can't cope with this!" springs to mind, many of us become completely fused with it and do not even try to cope.

Using the same parlance, the practice of producing an inner distance is termed "defusioning", and is very helpful in such instances. This allows us to recognize the thought for what it is – a thought not a fact. From the self-limiting thought "I definitely cannot cope with it" we can shift to an awareness of what we are experiencing right now: "I am having the *believed thought* that I would not be able to cope." We cease to transform a fear into a belief which we subsequently use to limit our responses to life.

What we have described to this point is how we relate to our experience in our day-to-day life. We are driven by certain behavioural patterns:

* attachment to what is pleasant
* aversion to what is unpleasant
* boredom or indifference to what is neutral

When we drop down onto the cushion to practise mindfulness we will experience exactly the same patterns; we become aware of problems, difficulties and we notice the reactions of our "automatic pilot". But whilst we are there, we can see with greater clarity just how we react to pleasant, unpleasant and neutral experiences. We have the chance to learn directly something about ourselves comfortably positioned on the cushion. Learning in this way, in our daily practice, is very safe. It is here we can create our own laboratory – a microcosm, a safe environment for our learning. Afterwards, we can transfer our insights and newly gained skills into our daily life – our macrocosm – to a life more mindful, more healthy.

Some traps, difficulties and disturbances

Mindfulness is used today in hospitals, organizations, schools and even the military as it has been for 2500 years in monasteries. By practising mindfulness consistently and continuously you will reveal thoughts and ideas more readily and have greater internal clarity. Even if you are still brooding a lot, you won't need to drive around the same block seven times, but you may be able, after the second time around, to slow down the worrying mind. Do not let yourself be kidnapped by your own thoughts any more!

When we are able to clean the dishes without ruminating at the same time over a thousand other things, we are on the road away from brooding. And we are also better protected against mental disorders such as depression or burnout.

There is no more promising way than mindfulness to learn how to deal with these obstacles, to pacify the war within. We will now explore some of the most common blockages raised about practising mindfulness by clients and participants at London Meditation and experienced by ourselves too.

"Am I practising mindfulness correctly?"

As soon as you have started your practice – no doubt highly motivated and committed to gaining all of the benefits – you will encounter the war within your body and mind. You may ask yourself questions such as: "What am I doing here?", and "What is going on?" You have been seeking relief and rest and instead you discover turmoil inside your body and mind.

Maybe at this point the first of a series of doubts arises, starting with "Am I doing it right?" You ask yourself this question because, for example, you were falling asleep during your first practice, felt uncomfortable during your first body scan, suddenly became aware of tensions everywhere in your body, you lost concentration. But this is exactly the nature of mindfulness. It lets us experience what is going on in our body and mind, allowing us to become aware of these events, to recognize them and enable us to continue observing them. *There is nothing right or wrong* with your first experiences. Mindfulness practice is not for enjoyment or entertainment, it is not even necessary that you like it – just that you do it.

Saying that, you will remember that mindfulness in fact is not doing something with intention or purpose; it is being in the here and now and without intention but with full attention to what is. Another question might be…

"How do I find the best conditions to practise in?"

Once we have discovered that *whatever happens* during our mindfulness practice is okay, we find another threat to disturb our introspection – external conditions.

The first of these may be the space we decide to use for our mindfulness practice. If you can avoid it, we do not recommend that you use the room you sleep in, or your bed. It is an environment you associate with sleep, and the atmosphere of the whole room is imbued with a sleep energy – it does not support the calm, but alert and fully awake state which is appropriate for mindfulness observing.

Ideally, we need to find ourselves a space which is conducive, with few or no intrusions from outside. But what if there is no such place available? The physical space in which you practise should at least be somewhere that you feel safe, but not being able to fulfil the ideal conditions should not deter you from practising.

What happens when there is noise from the street outside such as traffic, a train or airplane, a barking dog, a tweeting bird, a crying infant or an audible heating or cooling system? When we start our practice in a relaxed manner, these sounds will be there and we will be aware of them. We allow them to be, because there will be always something coming into our awareness, attracting or disturbing us. We acknowledge them and let them be. There is no need to follow them or to judge them because they exist. We allow them to be where they are and come back with our attention to the subject of our observation.

"My body hurts when I'm practising!"

When we notice in our formal meditation practice that the body is becoming uncomfortable, or we notice areas of tension in our body, questions arise about how we deal with these. Unpleasant bodily sensations arising is commonplace in formal practice, particularly in longer ones, and we will notice this again and again. So when you do notice this, you have two different options.

One option is that you allow yourself, very slowly and deliberately, to slightly move your body. This means that you are taking action on purpose, and are moving your body, but this time, instead of moving on automatic pilot, you are noticing and observing the movement itself. You are exploring the impact this movement has, particularly on the unpleasant bodily sensations you had noticed.

Mindfulness for relief

As an illustration of how mindfulness can be useful in addressing physical irritation or pain, here is an anecdote from one of the author's own experiences:

"Before I gave up smoking in 1999 I was a very heavy smoker: a couple of packets a day, mostly menthol flavoured cigarettes. This often resulted in tremendous headaches, especially in the evenings. A wise man and fellow meditator reminded me not to fight against the pain, or to avoid it by swallowing a paracetamol, but rather sit with the headache and hold it as a bodily sensation in awareness. It might seem like a crazy idea, but it's sound logic for a meditator...

...So I used these situations to sit with the pain and to witness it. After a couple of sittings I finally received the insight: that the headache was nothing else but my body's outcry of 'what are you doing to me, stupid?'

The moment this insight reached my consciousness the headache dissolved. But the insight worked on. It finally convinced me to give up smoking, which I did in 1999.

And now, as a non-smoker, if for whatever reason a headache arises, I understand it as a knocking on the mind from the inside. Then I can sit and hold it in awareness. And nearly every time I can see where it comes from and it vanishes. There is no need to take my word for it. Try it: find out for yourself whether it works or not!"

Moving during a formal mindfulness practice is not a crime, *as long as we are bringing awareness to the movement itself.* Then it becomes part of our practice. So this is the first option we have when unpleasant bodily sensations arise in formal practice. We start moving on purpose, observing the movement, and noticing the impact the movement has on our body.

The second option is to adopt a completely different approach. As we discussed earlier, we usually wish to get rid of unpleasant experiences, so we generally want to push these experiences away. However, we can choose to purposefully move our attention *towards* what is unpleasant in the body. This is a conscious decision and in itself might be challenging since we are moving our attention towards what is unpleasant.

We investigate the nature, the texture, the intensity of these unpleasant sensations in the body. As best as we can, we hold these unpleasant bodily sensations in our awareness; holding them with kindness and compassion in awareness. Without trying to change anything, just noticing, witnessing and holding them in our awareness, and seeing how they unfold over the next few moments or seconds.

"And my mind goes on and on!"

The nature of the mind is to produce thoughts. There is nothing wrong with this. The real question is how we relate to the *activity* of the mind.

If we try to fight with it, to stop it, or empty the mind, then we are beginning to see the activity of the mind as something that is wrong and therefore in need of correction. This means that we are swiftly returning to a state of "doing" rather than "being".

Advanced mindfulness practitioners experiencing the mind and its activities have learned to see these manifestations of the mind in the same way that we perceive background music, or the sounds of the surrounding environment. They acknowledge the thoughts as present and they keep their focus on the observed subject or mindful task.

We can relate to what's going on in the background, when it becomes important to us, because we are aware of what is going on. But we also can decide to go on with our practice – undisturbed. It has become our *choice*.

"Formal practice requires time – which I don't have!"
Now we can hear a lot of you busy and stressed readers moaning: "But we don't have time for practising!" We know that many of the participants and clients of London Meditation

Mindfulness and awareness: a crucial difference

These are two states of consciousness that are easily confused. They are related, but they are distinct.

Mindfulness implies there is action of the mind. We purposely set ourselves to pay attention to our mind. We exert effort. Awareness is different. Awareness is devoid of any action. The mind is simply "aware" – there is no action here, only a collected and spontaneous awareness that just "sees". Here, mindfulness is the cause and awareness is the effect. We cannot practise or train the effect. We can only practise something that will cause it. We have to start with mindfulness, so that awareness may arise in us.

That sounds simple, but it is not easy and needs a commitment to practise. By practising, we are able to build our mental muscle and create the necessary support for this process of being aware, getting distracted, becoming aware of being distracted and coming back to our chosen practice. Or as Mark Williams has expressed it: "The positive thing about this practice is that wherever your mind may be, you can always start again in the next moment. The essence of mindfulness is the willingness to begin over and over again."

are also painfully familiar with tight deadlines, schedules and overpowering workloads. We do understand this concern. But mindfulness offers us the possibility of moving from struggling with these exhausting issues to getting back in control of our lives, of managing our resources and capacities by being aware of what realistically works for us and what works against us.

We can burn the candle of our lives at both ends and risk running ourselves down. So the question then becomes: "Can I afford *not* to set time aside for my own mental and physical wellbeing?" If we weigh up the **ROI** – our return on investment – of the time and effort to practise mindfulness, we will find ourselves richly rewarded: allowing us to take up the challenge and the opportunity to learn to live our life in the present moment; exploring this for ourselves, making our own experiences. The only time we truly have – the present moment – is the only time anyone ever has to perceive, to learn, to grow, or to change.

"Mindfulness is boring!"

This brings us to another issue, one which appears to be the opposite of lack of time – boredom. Boredom is always a sign of inattention. The mind wanders around aimlessly. Nagging thoughts often arise such as: "What *am* I doing here, wasting my time?". And so on.

Try to remember that there was a time in your life when you welcomed change. As babies we were happy at the point when a wet nappy was removed and replaced with a dry one, changing us from a miserable crying infant back again into a lovely and curious baby ready to conquer the world. The world was full of new experiences, our bodies changing and acquiring new skills and our understanding of the world growing and transforming our relationship to it.

But our attitude to change is different in adulthood. Now we like what we already know and we stick to it even when it is not really helpful or healthy. What is known to us gives us the feeling of being safe – we are in our comfort zone. What we do not know creates doubt or even worse – fear. Most of us don't like changing what we know for something we don't.

But mindfulness makes us aware that life is a process of constant change. Change is reality. No wonder our minds are displeased as we progress in our mindfulness practice and become more and more aware of this constant change. And because the purpose of mindfulness is to become.aware of this impermanence, this fluctuation, without judgement and intervention, the mind believes that its role is to protect us. It employs all of the means at its disposal to pull us away from our "purposeless" and "dangerous" venture. So it generates feelings of boredom or restlessness, leading us to guilt and self-reproach about our engagement with mindfulness.

This is not helpful and it does not make sense. But the moment we become aware of this intervention by the mind, it is up to us to decide how to respond. We can choose either to run away from this eye-opening encounter with our self, or to embrace it by coming consciously back to our practice and allowing the chattering mind to be firmly in the background.

"I experience all sorts of irritations when practising!"

Another obstacle to practising when following the guidance in a recorded practice is a dislike for the voice of the facilitator. Sometimes it is the pitch and tone of the speaker, the terminology used, or just the facilitator's way of speaking. Whatever it is that we believe we cannot stand, this is no reason not to practise. There are so many recordings of the body scan and other guided mindfulness meditations on the market with so many different voices that it should be possible to find a recording that does not irritate you and supports your practice.

It is also worth considering using the experience of listening to a voice that you find less attractive as a way to work with negative emotions. You could do that by being genuinely curious; accepting these negative thoughts or feelings non-judgrmentally as a here-and-now experience which provides a compelling example of a different stance towards negative emotions.

In this way, you may also become aware at which point these negative emotions arise and if they are constant or fluctuating, how long they last and if other thoughts, feelings or bodily reactions are also drawn into this experience. Once again you have the opportunity to become aware of the reluctance of the mind to allow you to learn about yourself; its desire to sustain the old habits of avoidance and of trying to escape from negative emotions.

We say "Good Luck", because our experience shows that negative emotions will come and go and mindfulness can allow us to understand our negative emotions rather than battling with them. From this understanding, you can learn to live with them in a less haunted way.

"I find myself wanting to do other things when practising!"

Another type of obstacle or barrier we encounter in our formal practice is when pictures or feelings are arising about desires we have. This may be thoughts like:

* It would be nice to be with my partner now
* I would love to be on holiday now
* Walking with my dog would be great
* I would like to be cooling down in the swimming pool

Maybe we even taste the flavour of ice cream, fresh strawberries or a refreshing drink in our mouth. Well these are yearnings for things, events or places but they are, in this moment, just mental events and not reality. They are another mechanism used by the mind to get us out of our journey to ourselves.

What we do is to acknowledge that we have these desires and leave them on the periphery, recognizing them for what they are – thoughts or emotions. We let them pass by like clouds in the sky, birds on their way through the air or ships on the coastline and we continue with observing, witnessing, being aware.

"I feel sleepy when I try to practise!"

With mindfulness comes calmness and calmness allows relaxation. Given how exhausted many of us are, it is only natural that when we experience relaxation, our body uses this possibility to get the necessary rest to refuel our biological batteries. Those of us who suffer from sleep disturbances or insomnia are always happy when we get a refreshing nap or even better a good night's sleep. So in general there is nothing wrong with falling asleep.

It may be a welcome side effect of mindfulness practice that we become more and more relaxed but it is not the purpose, or intention, or goal of mindfulness. Sometimes too, it is a trick of the mind to allow this kind of sleepiness and drowsiness to arise in order to avoid the journey inside of us. Therefore, the real issue is how to relax *in* awareness.

Mindfulness is not falling asleep but *falling awake*! In this state, the body relaxes (and maybe even the mind) but we are still awake and indeed *more* alert and open because of this relaxed condition. Remember formal practices such as the body scan are more about finding our way to reconnect with our self, irrespective of whatever comes up   pleasant or unpleasant.

When we are too relaxed we fall asleep, when we concentrate too much, we feel tight and tense. It is important to find a good balance between relaxation and concentration, because both abilities are prerequisites for mindfulness practice.

"I am sceptical about the benefits of practising!"

The mind has no interest in being mindful. So it produces all kinds of different thoughts (desires, aversions, etc), and the emotions consequent on them, to take us away from this moment-to-moment experience.

You may be sceptical about the practice, the guidance or even the mindfulness teacher in a meditation class. For example, people who have attended a mindfulness class sometimes come out frustrated by the experience:

* I tried so hard but didn't get it
* It doesn't work for me

And sometimes they come up with the idea: "I think I need more discipline!" It is important to notice that these are all just states of mind, this time expressed as unfulfilled expectations. What is it that people are expecting from mindfulness? Are they looking for a mental painkiller, a neurological remedy, a stress buster, a magical cure? Well, they may experience some of the benefits of those things, but mindfulness is actually nothing of the sort.

When we talk about practising with commitment, we are talking about "non-doing" and not striving for goals or outcomes. We are talking about putting the emphasis on "being", about allowing things to be held in non-judgemental awareness, exactly as they are in this moment.

All of these phrases express concepts essential to mindfulness practice; that such practice involves letting go of the idea of fixing or changing things; that it is not about avoidance or

After the formal mindfulness practice

Once we have completed our mindfulness practice for the day, we should take a moment to reflect on what we noticed. Perhaps we noticed that we were feeling really stressed or angry or particularly calm today.

Or maybe we noticed that our thoughts were all over the place and that we were having trouble staying in the present moment. One thing is key: remembering to practise regularly, but always being accepting – however the practice went.

escape; it does not enhance, nor transport you to somewhere different in this moment. This is particularly relevant when the subject of the practice may give rise to emotions.

With emotions it is sometimes best to allow them to change themselves. Instead of trying to change them we simply observe them in the broad light of awareness, seeing them with greater clarity and holding them in awareness until they dissolve by themselves. Remember – they are transient, they will never *ever* last forever.

Returning to mindfulness

The direct awareness of present perceptions is one of the foremost wonders of being human, enriching our life beyond measure. Yet in our ordinary mode of living, we exist somewhere below the level of mindfulness, and do so at a largely unrecognized but terrible cost. Mindlessness shortens and impoverishes our life, shortens it in the sense that we experience less when we are not mindful. Impoverishes it in the sense that what we do experience remains less vivid, less alive, less real to us than it could be. Mindfulness is the authentic state for a human being: a relaxed, open awareness of our inner and outer perceptions in this moment.

While mindfulness is the birthright of all humans, to our great misfortune we sell it off cheaply. We spend the vast majority of our time unmindfully, our awareness passively collapsed to some tiny fraction of the whole, drifting along in a passing reverie, captured by anger, envy, lust, boredom, fear or greed. Our lives go on without us. Time passes us by, leaving us unmoved, unfulfilled and unaware, in a waking sleep.

Fortunately, the remedy for our situation exists. And it is a simple one, simple but requiring perseverance. Coming home again, bringing our awareness back to the riches of this one moment can be as simple as finding ourselves in awareness of bodily sensations, in the breath or in consciousness itself. We can readily enter mindfulness, at least for a moment or two. The more often we try it, the more we acquire a taste for it and the longer we are able to stay in it.

To re-enter mindfulness, we ground ourselves in our moment-to-moment awareness. This can serve as our foundation in the flow of experience. To practise mindfulness we begin by finding that comfortable home within ourselves. We repeatedly return to mindfulness until it becomes our normal way of being. In quiet moments we come back into basic mindfulness itself: unencumbered, without boundaries, featureless, whole, the background of all experience.

The enormous dividends of this simple practice of returning to mindfulness again and again more than repay our efforts. On a personal level, mindfulness dramatically enriches our quality of life and offers healing, meaning and wholeness, while serving as one of the fundamental components of presence. At the broader ecological level, mindfulness opens us to a profound connection with other people and all of life, as we will elaborate in Chapter 9.

But mindfulness needs effort, and for those dividends to accrue mindfulness needs to be pursued with diligence. By clearly seeing how things are in us, we avoid the trap of assuming we are already and even always mindful. Returning to mindfulness means coming home to ourselves again and again, moment by moment.

8

Meditations for daily life

In the first part of this chapter, we invite you to try a variety of exercises – short versions of formal practices. Implementing these exercises will support you to bring the learning you've gained in formal practice into your day-to-day life. Therefore it might be a helpful support for the informal practices.

The informal practices we would like to introduce you to relate to episodes and events you are likely to encounter in your daily life:

✱ Daily routines
✱ Mindful eating
✱ Mindful drinking
✱ Mindfulness (not only) for children

And finally we want to emphasize how we can relate differently to difficult moods, such as anger or fear, and highlight the importance of self-compassion in these situations.

The mind is like a megawatt searchlight, enabling you to see so much deeper into what you are gazing at. Ordinary concrete becomes a masterpiece. A blade of grass literally shimmers with the most delightful and brilliant shades of fluorescent green. The pretty becomes profound and the humdrum becomes heavenly under the sparkling energy of power mindfulness.

Ajahn Brahm

From Mindfulness, Bliss and Beyond

Short exercises

Mindfulness is something that we will ideally learn to integrate into all the moments of your life. These easy exercises are a great way to help you experience moments of mindfulness – brief awakenings, so to speak. All of them will support you in taking another step towards a more conscious experience of life.

Mindfulness vs. concentration

It is important to realize that there is a difference between mindfulness and concentration.

Concentration is of course a vitally important human faculty. It helps us to focus our attention on one thing or another and in this way it helps us to take command of what goes on in the mind.

But mindfulness is a step beyond concentration. Mindfulness is a state of awareness. It is *presence* of mind. Concentration is the tool we use to corral the mind to pay specific attention, to close the door on mental chatter. But it remains up to us to be present in the moment – to "show up now".

Exercise: one minute of breath awareness

This is an easy mindfulness exercise: one that you can do anytime during the day. We invite you to take a moment to try this right now.

* Find a way to measure the sixty seconds. Ideally this should be via some kind of alarm – perhaps the alarm clock function on your mobile phone – as you don't want to be distracted by having to check a watch

* For this minute, your task is to move all of your attention to your breathing. It's just for one minute, but sometimes it can seem like an eternity

* Leave your eyes open and breathe normally

* Remember, when the mind starts wandering off (and it will), return your attention to the breath

This mindfulness exercise is very powerful. It takes persistent practice before we are able to complete a single minute of alert and clear attention. It is important that we keep in mind that this mindfulness exercise is not a contest or a personal challenge. You cannot fail at this exercise; you can only experience it and learn from it.

You can practise this exercise many times throughout the day to restore your mind to the present moment and to bring it back to calmness and clarity. Over time, you can gradually extend the duration of this exercise into longer and longer periods. This exercise is the essential foundation of any mindfulness technique.

Exercise: counting the breath

This is a simple variation on the first breathing exercise. It is perhaps more of an exercise in practising concentration than it is in practising mindfulness. In this exercise, we stay attentive to the present by focusing on our breathing rhythm and we count the following complete breaths from one to ten:

* We breathe in and count one
* We breathe out
* We breathe in and count two
* We breathe out

…And so on up to ten.

If our mind is wandering off, we begin again, going back to one. For example, your train of thought might go something like this:

* One. Two. Three. Do I have to buy milk today?
* Oh, whoops, I'm thinking
* Time to start again with one.
* One. Two. Three. Four. This isn't so hard after all
* Oh no! That's a thought!
* Start again!
* One, two, three, four, five – now I've got it!
* I'm really concentrating now
* But that's a thought as well!
* Start again!

We need to remind ourselves again and again that this is an exercise in concentration and it is not a competition with ourselves. It is to make us aware and train our mental muscle, to develop the mindful skill of holding in pure awareness whatever we want to encounter – on purpose and non-judgementally.

Exercise: mindfulness cues

In this exercise, we bring our attention to our breathing whenever a specific environmental cue occurs. For example, whenever we hear the phone ring, or a new email announced, or a car horn outside, or a shout from the street, we promptly bring our attention into the present moment of our breathing.

So simply choose a cue that works for you. You needn't be in a static position for this. You can perform this exercise on the go. Perhaps you might choose to become mindful every time you look in the mirror or every time you open the door. The mindfulness cue could be every time your hands touch each other. It could be every time you hear a bird or see a child.

Using mindfulness cues is an excellent mindfulness technique designed to snap us out of the unconscious autopilot state and bring us back into the present moment.

Exercise: three-minute breathing space

The breathing space is an exercise that can be varied for different occasions and situations. This exercise comprises three stages, each lasting one minute. It is a technique that allows us to face whatever is arising in the present moment, including perhaps difficult and unpleasant experiences, in a different way. Instead of denying that they are present and trying to avoid them, it allows us to relate to such experiences more healthily. There is also an audio version of a three-minute breathing space exercise downloadable from the Rough Guides website.

The first minute

First comes awareness. We recommend that you bring yourself into the present moment by settling into an upright and dignified posture. (Though this could be in a standing position or a sitting position.) Choose if you want to have your eyes open or closed. Notice moment by moment what is most predominant in your awareness. What is your experience just right now in this very moment?

* Are thoughts present right now?
* Do you notice any emotions?
* Are bodily sensations most predominant?
* Be open to all the different inner experiences, without focusing on anything specific
* Acknowledge whatever is emerging and register your experience as it is – whether you like it or not

The second minute

In the second minute, we are breathing consciously:

* Begin to redirect your attention towards the breath in the abdomen as best you can
* Attend to each in-breath and each out-breath, as they ebb and flow like the waves of the ocean

Your breath is functioning as an anchor to hold you in the present moment; it allows you to make a transition into a state of awareness and stillness.

The third minute

Now we expand our field of awareness from our breathing; we allow a sense of our body as a whole being to become apparent.

* Sensing your body as it is; this includes being aware of any discomfort or tension in the body
* Allow yourself to gently move your attention to these difficult bodily sensations. If possible, breathe into the specific part of your body that is the source of the unpleasant sensations

- **Explore the impact this "breathing into it" has. Hold your experience in awareness. As best you can, open up to these unpleasant sensations and soften them by creating a sense of spaciousness around them**
- **Explore the impact of using mental notes – words repeated silently in the back of your mind. These might include:**

  It's OK!

  Whatever it is, it is okay!

  Let me feel it!

This breathing space enables us to leave our automatic pilot mode behind and come home to the here and now again. The key skill is to maintain our experience in awareness in the present moment – nothing more and nothing less.

Exercise: conscious seeing or listening

In this exercise, we choose an object on which to focus, allowing our attention to be fully absorbed by it. It may be a mundane everyday object, such as a coffee cup or a pen but we may also decide to focus on something more attractive to us, such as a flower, a tree, a candle or a beautiful panoramic landscape. We will be observing it, not assessing it, thinking about it or studying it intellectually. We are observing it for what it is.

Notice how quickly your mind fires off thoughts about the details of what it is you are perceiving – and starts to interpret them. But in this practice we simply notice the object as patterns of colour, shape and movement. And whenever your mind drifts off, or is elaborating stories about what you are observing, consciously bring your attention back to seeing the chosen object without any labels. This exercise is subtle, but powerful. By practising in this way, you will really start to sense what mindfulness is all about.

We can also practise conscious "observation" with our ears – listening – rather than with our eyes. Indeed, some of our participants find that mindful listening is a more powerful mindfulness technique than visual observation.

Whether watching or listening, the practice allows us to switch from the "doing" mode to the "being" mode, the destination we want to arrive at through mindfulness practice.

Informal practices in daily life

Informal practices can be useful in order to fit in with specific situations in our day-to-day life; with activities and functions we usually execute without any attention to the process of them. Because we do these things day after day we have lost our curiosity about these routine activities; informal practice allows us to re-encounter them and to become aware again of the uniqueness of these simple activities.

The task is always the same: observing what happens non-judgementally and on purpose, but without having any special intention, goal or purpose; bringing our attention fully to what we are doing right now with pure curiosity; and becoming aware of what arises or occurs.

Daily routines

Whatever your routines are in your daily life, you can bring a mindful approach to them. Here is a list of some of the phenomena you might typically experience in an average day, from the moment you first open your eyes in the morning.

Waking up

Be aware of:
* the fact that you are awake

* your first thought or feeling
* your breath
* how your body is getting out of bed

Taking a shower

Ask yourself:
* how does it feel to step into the shower cubicle?
* are there any thoughts, feelings or bodily sensations?
* how do you experience the feeling when the water touches the skin? Are the first drops of water hot or cold?

Be aware of:
* the sound of the water when it comes into contact with your skin
* the smell of shower gel, soap or shampoo
* the relationship of soap, hand and skin
* the sensations when the towel wraps the skin

Brushing your teeth

Be aware of:
* the tongue in relationship with the teeth, both before and after the cleaning process
* the encounter of the brush and the gums
* the taste of the toothpaste
* brush movements
* the water in the mouth
* spitting out the water

Shaving

Be aware of:
* the sound of the bristles when a hand runs over them
* the shaving foam meeting your skin
* the shaving process
* the water cleaning the remaining foam
* the skin afterwards
* the shaving lotion in contact with the skin

Looking in the mirror

Be aware of:
* your relationship to what you see

Drying your hair

Be aware of:
* your wet head and hair
* the sound of the hair dryer
* the first blow of the pressurized air
* the temperature of the air
* the relationship of hair, scalp and air
* the changing wetness and temperature of the hair

Interacting with other people

Be aware of:
* the fact that you are not alone
* what is said
* how it is that you initiate contact with others
* what you say while you are speaking

Commuting on the train, tube or bus

Be aware of:

* the environment where you are waiting (station, bus stop etc)
* people coming and going
* the travel conditions
* the people around you
* the smells, sounds and movements of others
* any touches or bumps you have with people or things
* your feelings and thoughts
* the weather conditions
* your body movements, posture and sensations
* changes in posture and moods
* the duration of moods and poses; how quickly they change

Concluding your day

Be aware of:

* the feeling that it is time to go to bed
* the transition from being upright to lying down
* your thoughts, feelings and bodily sensations
* the sounds around you
* the breath
* the relaxation process
* the transition from being awake to falling asleep

All of these short moments in life – maybe a few minutes each – are worthwhile and are important enough to warrant a bit more of your attention. You will also be surprised by how much you may discover by doing these routines mindfully. They may be transformed from being of little interest into events which are eye-opening, even shocking; everything is possible and don't forget: we only have to pay attention, observe, listen, feel, sense, nothing else.

And be creative! This list is not exhaustive at all, of course; if we are observing carefully, we will always find relationships and events in our lives worthy of a more mindful exploration, letting these reveal themselves to us naturally and in their own time.

We can practice anywhere – we can practice in places and at times when we are undertaking everyday activities. And those around us may not even recognise that we are doing anything unusual. For our formal practice, we set aside a specific amount of time and we create a supportive space. But the informal practice does not need any special arrangements: it makes the often-heard protest "I do not have time!" doesn't wash here at all.

Mindful eating

Another possibility for informal practice, and a potentially joyful one is mindful eating. Towards the start of this book, we talked about becoming mindful as if it were a physical journey into new lands. Well, you might wish to imagine now that we have been travelling for quite a while and that it's time for a treat. We've been holding off, waiting for the delicious taste of whatever comes to our minds: ice cream, a doughnut or some tempting strawberries?

* We take the first bite. Delicious!

* We take the second bite. It tastes great; though maybe a little less yummy than the first bite. But never mind. We

are scanning the landscape and something catches our eye: an animal, a person or a building. We are focusing on it, analysing and interpreting it and continue eating

* Suddenly we look down. Where did that treat go? Our fingers are sticky and there's still a trace of flavour on the tongue. So it must have disappeared down the hatch without us having properly enjoyed what we've eaten. A certain amount of disappointment and dissatisfaction set in. "That one just vanished! I'd better have another one..."

* Perhaps the internal weight-watcher turns up round about now to insist that one was enough. But the struggle over the simple, biologically pleasurable act of eating has already begun

When we discuss issues like this with participants during mindfulness classes and training, almost every time it prompts a range of contributions about difficulties with food and eating, ranging from poor appetite, people having no time to eat, an embarrassed confession of an addiction to chocolate to the palpable misery of binging and purging.

How has it happened that food and eating have become such a common source of unhappiness? And why has it occurred in countries with plentiful food? The fundamental reason for our lack of balance with regard to food and eating is that we've forgotten how to be *present* as we eat. We eat mindlessly.

Food is not the problem

Fat cells are just trying to do their job, which is to store energy for lean times ahead or for famine. For most of our evolutionary history, starvation was one snowstorm or drought away. Our fat cells are there to help us survive! The digestive system is just trying to do its job, breaking down food, absorbing nutrients and getting rid of what's not needed. Even food isn't really the problem: while it's obviously not a good idea to eat nothing but high-fat, high-sugar, high-salt foodstuffs, food is instrinsically neither good nor bad in itself. Food is food.

The problem is not in the food, the fat cells or the stomach and intestines. The problem lies in the mind. It lies in our lack of awareness of the messages coming from our body: from our cells and from our heart. Mindful eating helps us learn to hear what our body is telling us about hunger and satisfaction. It helps us to become aware of what within the **body–heart–mind** complex is hungry and how and what is best to nourish it. Mindful eating is a natural and informative way of radically altering your experience of food.

How mindful eating works

Mindful eating requires paying full attention to the experience of eating and drinking – both inside and outside of the body. We pay attention to the colour, smell, texture, flavour, temperature and even the crunchy sounds of our food. We pay attention to the experience of the body. Where in the body do we feel hunger? Where do we feel satisfaction? What does half full feel like? What does three-quarters-full feel like?

We also pay attention to the mind. We "watch" to see when the mind gets distracted, when our attention wavers from what we are eating or drinking. We watch the impulses that arise after we've taken a few sips or bites: to grab a book, to turn on the TV, to call someone on our mobile or to browse the Internet. We notice the impulse and return to just eating.

The old habits of eating and not paying attention are not easy to change. Don't try to make drastic changes. Lasting change takes time and is built on many small changes. We will start simply.

Hints and tips for mindful eating and drinking

Let's try to take the first four sips of a cup of hot tea or coffee with full attention. Imagine that we feel the cup on our lips. Every moment we are expecting the hot liquid pouring in our oral cavity; there is temperature, taste and a subsequent bodily sensation; it is either pleasant or unpleasant. We are savouring it for a moment and then we are swallowing it. There is again the temperature when it runs down our throat... and the aftertaste when it disappears into our stomach; the remembrance of what has been.

If you do want to read and eat, try to alternate these activities; don't do both at once. Read a page, then put the book down and eat a few bites, savouring the tastes, then read another page, and so on.

At family meals, we might perhaps ask everyone to eat in silence for the first five minutes, perhaps thinking about the many people who have been involved in getting the food to our plates here and now. We should try to eat at least one meal a week mindfully: alone and in silence. This may require a bit of creativity if you live with other people, but do try to find occasions when this is possible. Could you find a quiet spot somewhere in your office building or environs – perhaps in a nearby park?

Eventually, once you have properly developed the ability to be with yourself, you will be able to find an appropriate place anywhere and at any time you want it – undisturbed in the midst of our frantic world.

Exercise: mindful eating

This mindful eating exercise may be especially pleasing to some because it involves chocolate. But there is no need to fear; it is waistline-friendly as we really only need one piece of chocolate – or two if you want to do a comparative study.

You will need one or two squares of chocolate (or alternatively, two chocolates or a small chocolate bar cut in half).

Examine the unopened chocolate

Be aware of:

❋ The packaging

❋ The smell that comes through the paper

Feel the anticipation

❋ Open the bar/box

❋ Watch how the wrapper comes away; how it crinkles and crackles; and then reveals the chocolate within

Notice how the chocolate looks

❋ Observe the texture, the aroma and any imperfections made during its manufacture

❋ Break off a square and breathe in the aroma

❋ Look at it: the sheen, any decoration on it, the way it has broken off from the bar. (Note: You don't have to *stare* at it, just look at it for what it is)

❋ Observe how it feels in your hand

❋ Smell it again, the sweetness of it, its chocolate-ness

Take a bite, or place the square in your mouth

❋ Feel the sensation as it rests on your tongue

❋ Savour the flavour of it – what can you taste?

❋ What is the texture like?

❋ Roll it around in your mouth and pay close attention to the changing texture and taste; notice how it starts to change from what was once solid

❋ Continue focusing on all the characteristics until the chocolate has been eaten and all that remains is the lingering aftertaste

* Did you enjoy it?

* Can you feel the flavour that is left in your mouth?

The comparison step

* Take the second piece of chocolate, but eat it how you normally would. Which for most of us means to pop it all in your mouth, give it a couple of chews then gulp

* Do you experience any difference?

* Did it taste the same?

* Did it taste worse?

* Did it taste better?

We have tried this experiment with various different people. All said it tasted better the first time. One participant even thought they were different types of chocolate.

Mindful drinking

When you visit the Penthouse, the home of London Meditation, you might be surprised to notice our small shelves containing sophisticated wines – surprised because you might not expect to find alcohol in a place of mindfulness. The explanation is simple. Mindfulness does not mean a strict ban on every kind of pleasurable substance; it means being aware of their effects and enjoying them responsibly, in a healthy way.

We know that people experiencing ongoing unmanaged stress tend to develop unhealthy habits, which include drinking too much alcohol or caffeine, overeating, smoking and the like. These bad habits undermine health as much as the stress that triggers these behaviours.

By contrast, an effective, mindful approach to stress management includes an appreciation of well-prepared and nutritious food and a glass of wine to complement the meal if you'd like. While it is not necessarily the mental picture conjured up by the word mindfulness, time simply spent with people you love, or the appreciation of a good cigar after a delicious dinner in front of a cosy fireside can be very mindful. If, that is, our attitude is the appropriate one, regarding the experience as being nurturing of ourselves.

The mindful art of experiencing wine

First, make sure not to overfill the glass. If your glass is too full, it prevents the perfume of the wine, its 'bouquet', from filling the nose. Much of the pleasure of drinking wine is in the smell, which is the greater part of taste.

So, pour just one or two fingers high into the glass and swirl it round a little before sipping. The wine's aroma will escape from the glass and its flavour will develop with the addition of air brought in by the swirling.

You can enjoy the beauty of the wine's colours particularly well if you spread out a white napkin on the table or have a white tablecloth. Allow your eyes to rest on the colour, gazing not staring, drinking in the colour with your eyes.

Maybe you are already becoming aware of body sensations such as your mouth watering, the appearance of saliva in the oral cavity provoked by the inviting colour and the promising smell of the wine. Hold this sensation in your awareness exactly as it emerges at this moment, for a moment.

As you have all the time in the world, you will take a conscious, small, first sip while smelling the more concentrated notes in the glass. You will be sipping in a way that brings yet more air into the wine. For once, ignore the idea that it is impolite to slurp, and keep the wine moving around the different areas of the tongue for a while. You are tasting the wine, experiencing its structure, temperature and consistency and being open to, and curious about, what your taste buds disclose to you. Remember – you have all the time in the world, because you have allowed yourself this "me-time"!

Then there will be the moment, when you enjoy the velvety feel of the wine slipping down your throat – slowly and consciously – and its aroma moves up from your throat into the back of the nose. Hold this moment in awareness as undisturbed as possible. How does this feel?

* We imagine that we might feel lovely and relaxed, happy and appreciative of the carefully tended grapes and the caring winemakers who brought passion and expertise to the production of the wine

* ...and/or grateful for the company we are in if we are with others

These techniques for tasting wine are used by professional wine tasters and now that you have tried them, you will understand why! No more gulping wine just because you are stressed-out, please. You will miss all of its beauty and calming effects.

Mindfulness exercises (not only) for children

Wine tasting is definitely something for the grown-ups but this doesn't mean that there are no mindfulness practices which are also appropriate and very beneficial for kids. Nobody should force children to participate in any kind of meditative activity. So our advice is to invent games that have fun written all over them, rather than telling your child to sit down and contemplate "the moment" without moving for ten minutes.

Try games that don't have any buzzwords or phrases attached to them. You know, the ones we use all the time on our journey here – such as "being present", "being aware", "being mindful". This is drivel to most kids and sounds like instruction – not something fun to do. Instead, try the mindful exercises we suggest below, and then develop your own ideas. Innovate!

Exercise: stroking the dog (or cat)

Provided you have a peaceful, non-aggressive animal, this is a winner!

* Encourage your child to stroke the animal, first with his or her eyes open for a minute...
* ...and then with their eyes closed for a minute
* Suggest to them that they stroke slowly and gently
* Ask them what the fur feels like in each situation

With eyes open, the fur is likely to just feel like the fur of the animal; with eyes closed, the imagination homes in on the texture – interpreting the cat's fur as wool, carpet, a bath mat and all kinds of other things that kids tend to imagine.

This game is fun because it promotes affection toward nature, stimulates the imagination and teaches the child to appreciate the beauty of that moment, and the connection with the animal.

Exercise: roaring in the wind

Next time it is windy in the garden or park, or if you are on a windy beach by the sea, stand facing the wind with your child.

* Spread your arms out and ask your child to do the same
* Open your mouth and roar into the wind!
* Let the wind consume your face, hair and chest

This is so much fun – kids love the freedom of roaring and the idea of challenging the might of the wind. It is a great way to let loose naturally with your child in a primal game: an exhilarating mindfulness!

Exercise: watching ants

Ants are amazing, yet most of us don't know it because we are too busy killing them and sweeping them out of our homes.

Start by searching for some ants, maybe under a rock or near some spilt food or a tree in the park or garden. Once you've found them, provide the ants with some breadcrumbs. Then take a magnifying glass and let your child observe how amazing these creatures are. Watch them:

* working as a team
* carrying the crumbs back and forward
* assisting each other with the heavy load

There is absolute mastery in the way ants work and navigate difficult obstacles. Children will be thoroughly amazed. It is a valuable lesson in mindfulness (and not only for kids) when we appreciating nature in this way and recognize that ants, like humans, have a rightful, important place in the world.

How to work with difficult emotions

Emotions are the traffic signs in our life. They lead us, they warn us, they show us diversions and different routes and sometimes they even stop us. We need to be familiar with them and gain a deeper understanding of their value for us. To hold them in awareness allows us to identify the various aspects of these mood states.

A helpful mindfulness approach to becoming more and more acquainted with emotions begins with:

✳ Registering what is here

✳ Allowing what is here to be as it is, in this moment

✳ Simply holding it in awareness

These are the three aspects which offer us the possibility of accepting difficult emotions.

What does this mean in practice? Well, take a pause (and if you're not already seated, sit down). Notice what you are feeling right now. Whatever the emotion that arises – amusement, confusion, frustration, wistfulness, sadness – recognize the emotion and name it. And once the feeling is known to you by name, remember that all experiences, including feelings and emotions, are transient: they arise, last for a while and then disappear again.

The only thing we intend to "do" is to watch their coming and going with patience and a non-judgemental awareness. Watch them with an open mind and curiosity about the unique nature of any current emotion. You might become aware of its intensity, strength or other qualities. As best you can, open up to this feeling. There is no need to react or reject it, to suppress or to ignore it, and especially not to become hostile towards this emotion. It's much more important that you loosen up. By breathing into it, you can create a mental space around this emotion.

Imagine the situation as a laboratory, a place where you are able to find a workable distance from which to witness anger or fear or whatever is there. You are becoming aware that you are not the emotion, you are much larger than that, and can observe it in your own time. You are not dependent on this emotion.

When the emotion has a high degree of intensity, try to get closer to it – carefully and gently. If the feeling seems to become overwhelming, notice how your body is involved in this emotion. If possible, reconnect with your breathing rhythm for a few moments and when you feel strong enough again, come back to the still present emotion and explore it further. If you are patient enough, you will feel the emotional pain subside and there will only be a residual and temporary memory left.

So patience and openness to the outcome is the key to gaining this important knowing of impermanence. We want to offer examples (for anger and fear) that illustrate how applying this approach in our day-to-day life could work. A good way to start this is to wait until you feel you need a change.

* I must...
* I ought to...
* It's time to...

Of course, there are scheduled events we may have to attend to during the day. So it may be that we want to change something, not because we want to do something new, but want whatever is making us feel fed up, bored, irritated or depressed to end.

Anger is difficult to work with

Rage sweeps us away and before we know what has happened we are already upset; we don't notice what's been going on until hours later. But like many difficult challenges, recognizing and dealing with anger has great rewards. To start with, we may only be able to notice our anger when it begins to subside. This is okay. Any noticing is good!

So as we practise mindfulness, we can notice anger and name it. We can say "Anger is here!" Now we can witness what happens in our body to become aware where the anger is located.

* Look at your body and notice where the anger is
* It might be in your stomach, or shoulders, the muscles in your neck
* Consciously go with your breath into this part of your body to soothe and relax it

Anger may register first in the body as tension, a headache, or upset stomach. It may be picked up more readily in the mind. The following example addresses this.

The person who talks nonsense

Let's say we are sitting next to someone who is talking utter rubbish. It's totally opposed to everything we know to be true. We want to either straighten them out, or leave. They are unbearable!

So we give ourselves five minutes of trying to bear the unbearable (or as long as we can cope with!). With practice you will get better at this. Starting with your body, see how it feels. Check where the discomfort is. Some particular part will be carrying the strain: where is it? Now breathe into this part.

Find the name of the current emotion and then say it to yourself. Are you just bored? Or would it be better to call it anger or low mood? Say "Anger is there", or name whatever the emotion is. Now summon up every scrap of that emotion you can bear. Thoroughly expose yourself to it – after all, it's only for a few moments. Hold it in awareness.

When your five minutes are up, you'll find your mood has shifted at least slightly, maybe quite a bit. Do your five minutes with the unbearable and then make the change you want to make. But as you persist with this exercise you'll find yourself more at ease. You will no longer be as angry as you were, or at least you can calm down more quickly. Even your tolerance for the "idiots on the road" is better. Around the unbearable things in our life we develop a sense of humour, an ability to cope and make the best of difficult situations.

Moving on through this journey of mindfulness practice we will be able to come back to our moods more often, our constantly changing moods: now depressed, now amused, now excited, now angry and always changing. It's a dance. Mindfulness gives us grace; it's like having spent all our life hopping on our right foot only, never knowing that our left foot existed or we could move the weight. Suddenly we've got another way to move – we are no longer stuck with a one-legged hop!

Observing anger

You may be wondering about the moral position of anger. Isn't it wrong to be angry? But by noticing it, by holding it in awareness and not trying to ignore it we are much less likely to leap quickly to act on it, or make judgements based on it.

We are often so wrapped up in thinking things such as...

* What should I do?
* Am I right to be feeling this?
* Whose fault is it?

...that often we forget to notice the simple fact that we are angry. Of course it's not good to lose our temper and shout, and it is, generally, very counterproductive. Violence, bodily harm, murder, war, genocide, rape and child abuse, all of them arising from anger and fear, are a world-wide blight. All over the world we have police, law-courts, prisons and armed forces established to deal with the consequences. But putting this right can only happen when each of us can address anger in our own hearts and acknowledge consciously to ourselves: "There is anger here". But in addressing this, we will be very tender with ourselves, just as we would be with a small child.

As we learn – through mindfulness practice – to hold anger in our awareness, we are giving ourselves a chance to allow our anger a place in our life, giving it a value. It starts to take its rightful place, to come forward appropriately as an emotion without consequent reaction, and so we win these few seconds – the chance to make a decision, to act instead of reacting automatically. Those few seconds could be enough to prevent a war that now need not be fought.

To name fear is to welcome fear

The dark shadow of fear rises up. It may be a memory of childhood terror stirred into life by an event of today. A word spoken in a certain tone, a certain smell, the flash of water in a saucepan and suddenly we remember the buried event. It returns roaring into our mind and the fear with it.

Or it might be something more concrete that frightens us. Our job is threatened or we are dismissed. How can we support ourselves, the family? Or we might just have been told that our partner's car has crashed and we put down the phone as if it were a broken body.

So whether we are working with real and frightening events in our life or the fears that could more properly be called delusions or flashbacks from our early life, the feelings are just the same. When we are afraid and people tell us it is just our imagination, we are still frightened, but then we end up with double the disturbance. Our heart pulls back and hides like a cowering dog.

How can fear be handled?

When we are entering unknown territory, fear may well arise. Fear is an emotional expression of not knowing and therefore feeling insecure and anxious. We need first of all to acknowledge the fear in our heart – because fear and courage both live there. This is the country of knights in gleaming armour riding out fearlessly to face the enemy or more currently in computer games, full of warlords, orcs and Amazons, riding out to face the power of darkness invading the homeland.

Naming the fear is like welcoming the fear – greeting it, saying hello. It allows us to switch from fear to courage. In the example above, having just had a phone call about our partner's car crash, terrible things will be running through our mind – we will be imagining death, serious injury, disability… Our minds go into high speed when we are frightened or very angry: our body tenses up in the ancient fight or flight response.

Direct control is not possible in these circumstances, but we can sometimes take a moment to realize that we are frightened and our body is shaking. When we realize just how frightened we are, it's the first step. It allows the fear to be there.

When a scary thought arises, we experience the fear in our mind. This is a *real* mental event. When we feel the fear in our body then this is a *real* bodily sensation. Fear often starts in the mind and triggers a physical sensation. Remember – all our emotions are transient: they arise, stay for a while and vanish again.

If we now allow ourselves to have time to sit down for a moment and breathe with the emotion – hold it in awareness, stay in the present moment – our relation to the fear changes. All of this means: be consciously aware of what happens, non-judgementally and on purpose… We are able to become aware of what it is – an emotion, a brain-chemical reaction – instead of identifying with it and plummeting into the creation of a dramatic story. We work with the fear, by naming it as best as

Smiling is a technique

Smiling is a crisis technique (but it's good to do at any time!) – using our heart to smile. This is not a matter of "covering things up" or putting on a good face.

Allowing the fear itself to smile is a matter of being accommodating: you can allow your fear to crack open in a smile. Smiling is a technique taught by Thich Nhat Hanh, a world-renowned Buddhist monk and scholar, and it is employed in his community in Plum Village, France. We can use it with any deep and painful emotion and it's a good thing to do when things are very bad.

We consciously feel the grief, fear, anger or stress in our heart and then we allow the emotion to smile. How can this be done? We can do it physically – we simply ignite it by using our facial muscles and just smile! It heals the heart and fires up our courage. When we consciously switch from feeling the difficult emotion to the honest facial expression of smiling, the unpleasant fear cannot stay, because loving kindness to ourselves and the world around us will soothe our feelings and allow us to switch.

When, for example, we train people who work in a call centre to deal with their emotions after experiencing an angry caller, we encourage them to have a small mirror in front of them, where they can face themselves and smile at themselves before they pick up the phone again. And yes, it works most of the time.

we can, finding out where it lives in our body and breathing with it. First we allow the clarity to emerge as to what really causes the anxious feeling and then we name it. By practising choiceless awareness (see box in Chapter 14, p.258), sooner or later we will become aware what really causes the fear.

Very often, we will find that just spending a few moments with our fears, at the time they come up, is enough to make us feel different. Fear makes ghosts of us, empty shells, bloodless and withdrawn from life. It may paralyse us and leave us feeling out-of-control, at the mercy of our emotions. If the fear is an old one, it will take time and extra care before we can breathe the breath of life and see our courage return.

Relationships grow over time and that it is what we develop: a relationship to the fear. When we are able not to fight it, not to be anxious about the fear, but become able to hold it in awareness and be with the fear, our relationship to it changes. This change we *can* manage; it is under our control. It is our decision to fight or let go.

Even when we are unable to directly control our emotions, there is always the potential, the opportunity to switch from fear to courage. And we can start the transition with a smile.

Being ready for reality

Whatever type of life we are living, it will be enhanced by mindfulness practice. Mindfulness doesn't add anything, but we see the meaning of life more clearly through our mindfulness practice.

Jon Kabat-Zinn reminded us that we should not hold off weaving a parachute until the moment we jump from the plane. With mindfulness practice we are developing an open mind – one ready to sense – and what we are sensing is ourselves and what we hear is our life. When we have developed the skill of simply holding in awareness what is, as it is, we will be ready for whatever life holds for us. That means being ready for reality!

When we start our practice it doesn't matter what we are

like. We don't have to be good, or clean, feeling peaceful or "ready for meditation". We start our practice with an open mind, ready to listen, taking along whatever we may feel. Wherever and whatever we are is fine.

Curiously enough, many people who have practised mindfulness for a long time still feel like a beginner. We all still sit down on our cushion with a bunch of worries, addicted to things we think we should give up and worried about not doing things we had promised to do. It's always an effort. If we aren't making an effort then we aren't at the trailhead, the point where we set out again and again.

Some of the changes mindfulness brings us we will notice by ourselves. Some of them may not be noticed by ourselves. They will be spotted by our family, friends or colleagues: our character and identity changes. The practice of mindfulness puts us in touch. It connects. The results can be seen immediately and they also continue to grow with practice.

We will become more sure of who we are, more confident, more certain about things. We will be able to weather a crisis better. Our sense of humour will carry us through impossible situations and we learn to laugh at ourselves.

Making friends, forming relationships

By learning about ourselves and perceiving our own weaknesses we can form relationships with others more easily, because we feel an instant fellow feeling. People will report that we seem more approachable, more willing to listen and open to love. That's because we are approaching the genuine core of ourselves – our authenticity – and being authentic makes us more and more attractive to the world around us; authenticity is sexy.

Mindfulness often unlocks our creativity, or helps us move into different fields of creativity. Some of the mindfulness participants we have known have started painting, or writing music or coming up with new ideas about interesting things to do in their garden. They have started making delicious meals or have learnt to prepare food as they experienced it mindfully. With mindfulness too, we become more in touch with our emotions. A bubbling flow of creativity will burst forth as our body comes back to health and our emotional life comes alive again.

Some people come to mindfulness classes because of a particular problem, seeking help with their relationship difficulties for example, or because of a major illness. Sometimes the original problem can never go away. But when we are practising mindfulness, our relationship towards the problem changes, and it might be that we no longer have to fight with our suffering because we have learned to move around it, perhaps even to dance with it and importantly, how to live with it. This allows us to get out of the loop of misery and back on the road towards happiness and fulfilment in life.

Compassion

When we have gained, through mindfulness practice, the mindful attitude towards life – compassion – we will be dealing more gently, kindly and patiently with ourselves and others. Rather than judging or condemning, we open our heart to really listen and hold in awareness our own and other people's experiences. We will allow ourselves to feel other people's suffering. We love people, not for what they can give us, or because we need something from them, but because we are connecting and empathizing with them.

With a compassionate mind, we can bring mindfulness into our own life, whether it is by deliberately directing attention to our breath and senses at different times during the day, taking a mindful nature walk, or beginning a simple meditation practice. We might want to centre our attention on each in- and out-breath, noticing the length, quality and sensations of the breath moving in and out of our body, without trying to force or change it in any way. We may also begin to become aware of the times in the day that we operate "mindlessly" and on automatic pilot, our head so busy with plans and worries that we don't even notice what we are feeling inside or what is around us.

Through mindfulness practice we are developing an observing mind that watches our own daily experience, notices our automatic patterns and gently redirects attention to the present moment. This is the beginning of growing a "mindfulness muscle" to help us navigate the winds of change and stresses in our life.

Eckhart Tolle expressed it so eloquently with the words: "Always say yes to the present moment. We surrender to what is. Say yes to life – and see how life suddenly starts working for us rather than against us."

9

Mindful communication in relationships

Up to this point, we have been talking about our own personal growth process: the new relationship we are establishing with our mind, body and emotional experiences and, from this, the possibility of reconnecting with our innermost core. The results of this transformation will be noticeable to those around us. It will have consequences for our loved ones, our friendships, for our contributions to the groups we belong to and for anyone else we come into contact with.

When we connect with others we are communicating. So let's take a closer look at how we can bring mindfulness into that process. We call it, as you might expect, mindful communication.

Mindful communication

Have you ever had the experience, whilst talking to someone, that they are not really listening to you? They act as though they are, but it is quite obvious that they aren't. The irony is that they almost certainly *think* they are communicating with us. But on a profound level, we feel that we aren't heard at all.

Communication is something we all engage in on a daily basis, but because of the pace of our lives, conversations often become mere strings of formalities. Examples of communication at its most superficial can be found in the kind of exchanges we engage in when we enter a shop and the shop assistant asks us: "How are you?" The chances are that they are on automatic pilot; simply going through the motions required by their customer-greeting "script", as opposed to really being interested in how we are doing. Living mindfully isn't – as we have seen – just limited to meditation practice, but can be applied to every aspect of our daily lives. Including the business of effective communication in our day-to-day interactions.

Hearing versus listening

Hearing is not a choice. Listening is. Hearing is a sensory happening. It is not something that we do actively or consciously. Conversely, listening means that we are paying attention. To be attentive means consciously directing our attention towards the person talking to us. Our interest in, or attitude towards the speaker, will create the quality of our listening. In our day-to-day life there are innumerable instances where we find ourselves remarking to ourselves on things we have heard; plenty of occasions in which hearing is involved. But we are not really listening.

Let's say someone tells us that they will talk to us later. That's a phrase with a meaning that's obvious, right? A perfectly simple, innocuous phrase. But what does that "later" actually mean? Does it mean five minutes from now? Does it mean five hours from now? Or five days from now? Is that phrase even a polite way of conveying the idea that they have no desire to talk to us ever again? The possibilities of what that phrase could mean are in fact endless.

What do we hear? That that person wants to talk to us later. But was that really what the person meant? When we start making assumptions or interpreting, we may come to conclusions that lead instantaneously to a miscommunication.

One of the participants at London Meditation offered the following example of poor, non-mindful communication from her own life. She was talking to a friend about a problem and had poured her heart out to him. When it was the friend's turn to respond, his reply totally missed the point. It seemed to be more focused on him; it did not really address his friend's concerns at all. Whilst she recognized that her friend had good intentions, he was just not listening.

She thought back to what his initial reaction had been: she was a little frustrated because she could not see how her friend could have so misunderstood what had been said. She started to wonder if maybe she had not expressed herself clearly. However, as she reflected upon what her friend had said to her, she realized that her friend was listening to her from the stance of his own perspective on the world, without placing himself in our participant's shoes.

Her friend had responded by immediately trying to find something in his life that corresponded to what our participant was feeling, without truly understanding what that was. It was as though he heard only one word and entirely missed the rest of the sentence. That whole interaction is sadly exemplary, because it is such a common experience. We can probably all think of similar conversations in our own lives. Indeed, we can probably think of plenty of times when we have been that friend. It serves to underline the importance of applying mindfulness to our own communication.

Our habitual ways of reacting to people

We all have experiences of moments when we have to engage in difficult communication with others for various reasons. Do you have habitual ways of reacting in these moments? Perhaps one or more of the following will sound familiar to you.

We may have the tendency to ignore someone; or avoid them; or to talk with them only about specific topics. With those whose opinions are different to ours we may even become aggressive and confrontational. Or even worse, we might become passive-aggressive or start to identify ourselves as "victims".

Mindful communication means listening and speaking with openness, empathy and compassion. One dictionary definition of communication is "the imparting or interchange of thoughts, opinions or information by speech, writing or signs". This is a straightforward, technical definition, so there is no mention of openness, empathy and compassion. Indeed, if we observe any regular interaction between people, the form of communication will appear to fit the dictionary definition. But is this really the way we want to interact with others? Let's find out if there is a healthier way of communicating.

Aspects of mindful communication

When we start a conversation, it is best to become aware first of all of the following aspects:

* **With whom are we communicating?**
* **What is the content of the communication?**
* **What do we really want from the person or situation?**
* **What does the other person want?**
* **How do we feel during this time?**

We ask these questions to clarify the situation, our intentions and to get into contact with ourselves. And if we become aware of any thoughts that are occupying our mind that are not related to our current communication... we let them go. We are removing – as best as we can – any sense of judgement about the person we are talking with.

To listen to someone with a preconceived notion of who we think they are or what they are about to say, puts us at a disadvantage because we may miss what we could otherwise learn from them. If we become aware of a difficult communication with someone it might be helpful, in addition, to reflect on the following questions:

* What do we actually get from the exchange?
* What do they actually get?
* How did the difficulty arise?
* How do we feel during and after the conversation?

Essentially, we're putting ourselves in the other person's shoes. Experiences are relative, meaning that people react and see things based on how they view the world. In mindful listening, we put ourselves in the shoes of the person who is talking to us and try to see the world from their perspective.

We would like to give you an example from our own life experience. In the early 1990s, shortly after the reunification of the two parts of Germany, one of the authors of this book, Albert Tobler, was sent as a church officer (a deacon) to the eastern part – to the former German Democratic Republic (GDR). There, many people had been supporters of the state ideology, to greater and lesser extents. After all, the GDR was a declared socialist regime; Karl Marx, the father of socialism, had described religion as "the opium of the people", the "sigh of the oppressed creature". For a deacon – a representative of the Church – religion was the one and only salvation, not a drug. Somebody who lives in the belief that religion is a drug "has to be misguided" in the eyes of a convinced deacon and his dedicated ecclesiastic point of view. But when he sought to understand why they had supported it, he realized that they held the pragmatic view that the political structure in question benefited them.

He did not share their beliefs, and he disagreed with them, but that was okay. Understanding why they thought the way they did made working with people so much easier. Eventually it gave rise to a situation where it was possible to draw up plans and actions for the future cooperatively, and to realize those plans in a mutual endeavour.

Being open-minded and curious about why people have a different perspective pays off. Try it for yourself the next time you are struggling in a conversation – you may be surprised.

As the speaker we seek to be clear

Just because something makes sense to us it does not mean it will make sense to another person. The authors of this book have a friend who has a very strange sense of humour. Most of the time, it sounds like he is insulting us, but in reality he is not. We don't think he is aware of the impact of what he says: he is always amazed that people get angry at him, or feel hurt after speaking to him.

Hurtful words can sometimes cause deeper damage than physical pain, so we should choose our words consciously and carefully. Not everyone is willing to give us a second chance. A sentence uttered without thinking can end a relationship, or cause a person to lose their job.

As the listener we seek clarity

If the person who is talking says something that we don't understand, or which is not very clear, we don't assume anything

– but we ask them to clarify their statement. We often assume that the other person means one thing when in reality they could be talking about something totally different. There is nothing wrong with asking questions to render something clear, as long as we ask them with compassion.

We pause before we speak

When someone asks us a question, we shouldn't just immediately start talking. Ideally, we should take at least a few moments to pause and reflect on the question and on how we want to answer.

You might think that's impractical, and worry that the person you're talking to will grow impatient, or assume you aren't very sophisticated, or are unintelligent. But have you ever become impatient when someone you have asked a question of has been slow to respond? How did you feel? Perhaps you subsequently realized that this was because you are unused to someone taking time to really consider your questions.

Try taking the time to properly weigh up a friend's questions and statements next time you have a conversation; you may be surprised at how much people really appreciate it when you take their questions seriously.

We "walk the talk"

Often, when we talk to someone, we like to present a certain image. We want to appear as perfect as possible. We want the other person to warm to us and to think highly of us. Many of us try too hard to be something we are not and end up trapped into acting that way throughout the conversation. Or, even worse, throughout our relationship with that person.

The best thing we can do for ourselves is to be ourselves. That means *speaking our truth*. It does not mean we have to be rude or mean. We can speak our truth with compassion and kindness.

Here's an example from experience. We once found ourselves in the middle of a conversation with someone who was very critical of people who were not vegans. He had assumed, based on his own lifestyle, that everyone with an interest in mindfulness and meditation would be, at the very least, a vegetarian; it had not occurred to this individual that he might be talking to two non-vegans. We had two choices. We could either pretend to be vegetarian or tell the truth. To do the former would have been the easy option; we could simply have told a few little white lies – anything for a quiet life – and moved on. But we went ahead and told the guy the truth.

We were calm and told him that we understood his point of view. We shared with him our thoughts on the issue. We ended up having a really fantastic conversation and none of us had to raise our voice once. Nobody likes to be lied to; it's never worth lying about who you are.

Keeping your promises

In a similar vein, if you make a promise to someone – for example, that you will send them something by a particular date – be sure to keep your word. We earn a great deal of respect when we do so.

And last but not least, if we have no desire to talk to a person ever again, we should not say we will give them a call sometime. Whether it is in the context of business or in a romance or with friends, being honest in what we say goes a long way, for everybody concerned.

People will ultimately remember us for the right reasons if we "walk the talk". It is the foundation of trustworthiness and reliability. These are qualities that make us the people that others want to talk to, people to whom they will listen.

Qualities of mindful communication

In our everyday life we often experience the pressure of needing to be in two places at once; never really focusing on one thing at a time. We are very well aware that aspects of mindful communication may seem time-consuming, but if we want to be successful in whatever we do and if we want to have meaningful relationships, it is essential to have appropriate communications with people. The only way to gain peoples' respect is if we respect them. Engaging in effective communication is crucial to this; using mindfulness is one of the best ways to achieve it. Being fully present and attentive to the person we are communicating with is an essential part of mindful communication.

We all want to be heard and understood. Sometimes, in order to have someone hear and understand us, we have to hear and understand them first. For that to happen, the qualities of *interpersonal mindfulness* are necessary: openness, empathy and compassion.

Openness

Beginner's mind, permeability and psychological flexibility are all other terms used in mindfulness practice that mean the same thing as openness. Mindfulness practice involves gradually taking off all the pieces of our suit of armour – whether physical, intellectual or emotional. This requires trust, of course, and our bodies have memories too, so there is quite a time lag before the mind and body are ready to let go of some old wounds.

One of the most profound secrets of learning anything new is keeping what has been called (in a mindfulness context) a "beginner's mind". What is the beginner's mind? An important part of it is described very well by the famous Zen story known as "Empty Your Cup".

A university professor went to visit a famous Zen master. While the master quietly served tea, the professor talked about Zen. The master poured the visitor's cup to the brim, and then kept pouring. The professor watched the overflowing cup until he could no longer restrain himself. "It's overfull! No more will go in!" the professor blurted. "You are like this cup," the master replied. "How can I show you Zen unless you first empty your cup?"

Emptiness is openness – being free of expectations, free of assumptions and free of so-called logical thinking (rationality).

Empathy

It has been scientifically shown that mindfulness develops empathy as well as enhancing our capacity to be present in increasingly adaptable ways. Being mindful helps our own health, sense of purpose and wellbeing, but it also helps our relationships with our partners and friends. Mindfulness and empathy can be seen as basic elements of all relationships. They are excellent means by which to create resilience in ourselves and instil it in the people around us. Empathy – the ability to understand the mental state of another – can be learned and one learning path is through a practice of NVC: non-violent communication. (This is also referred to as compassionate communication or collaborative communication – but all these terms refer to the communication process developed by the American psychologist Marshall Rosenberg in the 1960s.) NVC often functions as a conflict resolution process. It focuses on three aspects of communication:

* Self-empathy, defined as a deep and compassionate awareness of one's own inner experience

* Empathy, defined as listening to another with deep compassion

✳ Honest self-expression, defined as expressing oneself authentically in a way that is likely to inspire compassion in others

Listening is a very deep practice ... you must empty yourself.
You have to leave space in order to listen ...
Especially to people we think are our enemies;
the ones we believe are making our situation worse.
When you show your capacity for listening and understanding,
the other person will begin to listen to you, and you will have a
chance to tell him or her your pain ... this is the practice of peace.
Thich Nhat Hanh, *Buddhist monk and peace activist*

Compassion

The synergy of empathy and the understanding that arises when we put ourselves in the shoes of the other person creates the quality of interpersonal mindfulness, better known as "compassion". This quality also generates a desire to ease the suffering of others. To activate this quality, imagine the situation and sensations as the other person is experiencing them. Presumably they have experienced disappointments, failures and losses during their life and some of these painful experiences have left deep wounds about which they may not want to speak. To say that we understand the other person's situation fully might be far-fetched, but sometimes just a hint – a mere glimpse of what they might be suffering – is enough to ignite compassion.

Why do we need mindful communication?

Mindfulness makes us aware of the source of our thoughts and emotions. Awareness also helps us to reduce the fragmentation of our self – to return to a sense of wholeness. This leads to a better appreciation of our self and creates increased self-esteem. It is only when we are feeling better about ourselves that we are able to make a positive contribution to society and to the world that we are part of.

Not only will this help us to feel more confident about ourselves, but it will also generate the desire and capacity to help others achieve the same confidence and self-esteem. But before this can happen, we have to overcome old and customary behaviours, patterns and belief systems.

If we are to be able to return some sanity to this world we share, we must hold ourselves accountable, develop compassion, exert healthy self-control and become more thoughtful in our words and deeds. Through practising mindfulness, we enhance our strength; our capacity to face our disappointments, fears and anger; and our ability to engage in the world positively.

Is mindfulness just escapism?

At this point, we are often challenged to answer the accusation that, given how the problems of the world are so complex, so vast and so frightening, practising mindfulness is somehow an avoidance of the responsibility to act in a more forceful fashion. Perhaps there's some truth to this charge. But perhaps thoughtful action, taken from a place of self-knowledge and patience, may be even more effective. At the very least it is likely that we will have less enmity in our lives.

It is human nature to believe that our efforts will eventually work. We keep trying, getting frustrated and then trying the same things again. We are certain that if we just try hard enough eventually the right combination of effort and timing will produce the results we are looking for. But do they?

What if our ideas about how to improve life are wrong? This may be a difficult idea to take on board, so let's pose the question even more simply. Which of the following would work better in your own life?

* Trying to change someone's point of view by arguing, posturing, persuading and manipulating

* Responding without trying to influence the outcomes for someone, living from a place of mindfulness of our own life and allowing the other person to do whatever they want

You may think that the second option is, effectively, giving up – not doing enough and being apathetic. But look around you. Are things working? Everyone is trying so hard to stay afloat, keeping abreast of the news, discussing what someone in power should be doing, lamenting what has gone wrong with the world and arguing about whose solutions are correct.

We can help others, but we must begin by focusing on ourselves. In nature there is an intrinsic progression that allows one life to affect change, without doing anything but caring for itself. You'll never see a flower trying to improve a distant field. It simply thrives and allows the wind and insects to carry its seeds, touching and affecting other living things along the way.

Focus on our own life. Remember the informal practices. Is mindfulness a world solution? It seemingly has nothing to do with public health, the economy, world hunger or climate change. But what if it did? Could mindfulness ever begin to elicit massive change?

Becoming more mindful will help us to notice things in the world that have never occurred to us. Our actions will come from a richer place; a calmer place, where inspiration and positive change flourishes for us and everyone around us. Try it. Let's see how it feels.

Mindfulness and relationships

If we are applying mindfulness specifically to the conduct of relationships, we can see it gives us an opportunity to enhance joy, compassion and connectedness. There are some ways mindfulness practice can enrich our relationships.

Meditation promotes relaxation and neutralizes the stress response. Being mindful of our breath and body can be emotionally and physically relaxing; it provides a buffer against chronic stress. It allows us to "just be" with what is; it calms the constant flow of thinking and emotional arousal that may follow stress triggers. As stress builds, so can agitation and conflict. Mindfulness can be a shared activity preventing conflict from arising at all. Mindfulness increases compassion for and acceptance of our partner – or those we live with.

We all have quirks, habits and qualities that can get a little annoying. When we are around someone day in and day out, it's important to develop a flexible and non-judgemental outlook! When we can accept the peculiarities and apparent squeamishness of our partner about certain things, those trivial problems no longer lead inevitably to discord. Mindfulness can help us be more objective and less reactive about these issues.

Mindfulness improves our ability to cope and function in different domains of life. It is a "way of being" as opposed to a specific skill. When we apply the insights and new skills gained from practising mindfulness to our day-to-day life, it makes our work, leisure and family responsibilities more pleasant and tolerable. It leads us to greater engagement in

Mindfulness and arguments

We can tell there's a storm brewing in our relationship. Our partner looks angry – we can see it. We know he/she is getting close to the boiling point. What do we do? Do we leave? Do we brace ourselves for the fight that's coming? Do we attack first?

We don't have to do any of these things. Instead, by being mindful of what's going on with our partner, we can learn to avoid arguments. Being mindful can help us to avoid fights and diffuse tension. How? Mindfulness can be used to help bring our attention to the situation before it escalates. The easiest way to bring our partner's attention to what we see is to simply comment on what we're noticing on the outside. We might say: "It seems as if you've grown quieter over the past few minutes"; or "I notice you've started pacing".

Our purpose is only to say out loud what we see or hear our spouse doing. It's crucial that we allow for the fact that we really don't know what's going on inside our partner. If we asked us to guess about the underlying cause, we would become an evaluator – and we all know how well *that* works. Be sure *not* to say "you seem to be getting upset," because that comment is a guess about their feelings inside. Unbelievably, people aren't grateful when you comment on that!

Instead of commenting on what we think our partner's emotional state is, make our remark about his/her behaviour on

momentary pleasures, greater clarity in our thinking and improves our capacity to cope with unpleasant events. For example, we may develop partner-focused loving kindness, learning to be mindful of daily pleasant events and improving intimacy through mindful touching and eye-gazing.

Intimacy – sexual intimacy specifically – requires the establishment of safety and comfort. When we are kind, caring, pres-

the outside, as if we're opening a door and inviting him/her in. Remember, however, that they will only enter or talk about it if they want to. We should think of it as narrating what we're witnessing, like a reporter. Keep in mind, however, that we're not a reporter who's uninvolved; we are this person's partner, so we must present our comment with kindness, curiosity and love. This is why our observation is followed with "tell me about what's going on for you?" This is a way of asking in a gentle, curious and non-demanding way, "do you want to talk about it?" It is done with support and caring.

It's important that we don't:

* jump to conclusions
* make assessments
* comment on what we think our partner's state of mind is, or react with judgment

The key here is to try something different in the way we notice and support, our partner. Being mindful by making gentle observations about our partner and asking him/her about it can give us the chance to step back, stop our own emotional responses and help avoid confrontation. We are opening the door for improved communication with less conflict. But always being accepting – however things went.

ent and attentive during sex, everyone has a better time. So the next time we want to spice up our love life, we should add a little sugar to the loving kindness and watch what happens. After all, even the Bible says, "The desire of a man is his kindness."

To sum up, mindfulness can improve our day-to-day relationship happiness, our ability to manage stress and to live compassionately – even whilst arguing with a loved one.

Mindfulness in groups

Common sense tells us that social gatherings are the last place to practise mindfulness; so crowded and noisy, so much stimulation, so much "mindlessness" all around. But have you ever tried it? You might find you arrive at another point of view.

Let us imagine the following scenario. More than twenty of your friends and associates have gathered together. Some of them you have more connections with than others. Many of them you only get to see once a year. Each new encounter offers a chance to observe the mind at work:

* How much do I really listen?

* How often and how fast do I judge the things people say?

* How quickly do I decide "I like this conversation"? Or alternatively "this person is boring"?

* How many "stories" from the past do I bring into each interaction?

* Am I preoccupied by, for example, what so-and-so said to me five years ago and which I still haven't forgiven? Or, say, the memory of a heartfelt conversation that once brought the two of us close?

* Who do I choose to speak to and who do I ignore?

* How does it feel right now in my body? Am I tensing or relaxing? What is the emotion?

Many of the above will doubtless sound familiar to you. There is so much to process in a matter of seconds. The trick is to catch the thoughts before they have a chance to get formed into words or played out as actions. There is joy to be derived from this, not just insight: joy from being more present and more kind. In the scenario we have laid out, there is only us and them, these near-strangers whom we will probably not see for another year or so. And from our point of view, the experience should not be about us, but about them and what they are saying. If we are truly mindful, we can feel the impurities of our own mind wash away, leaving our hearts free to meet them.

It is really extraordinary to go into a social situation after having had a mindfulness practice and to notice how much easier it is to interact with everyone. It is often remarked upon by participants in our eight-week programmes (as described in Chapter 10) when we have a celebratory drink or meal after the final session.

Mindfulness on its own does not cause any transformation; only insight can do that – the insights brought about by mindfulness. This is a fine, but important, distinction. These insights can be big or small, but they all do the same thing – they change our perspective. We stop seeing things in a confused way and we start seeing them with greater clarity.

Mindfulness gives us the energy to change our perspective; it is a prerequisite, but is not in itself enough for transformation to occur. To put it another way, mindfulness is temporary, while insight is forever.

Our emotions and social interaction

Just what are the psychological factors that cause problems with social interaction? Factors such as fear of rejection, humiliation, loneliness, loss of control, feelings of inferiority or superiority are frequently implicated. These mental formations cause all sorts of reactive patterns which tend to kill conversations and make things awkward. We may hope that mindfulness allows us to get to a point where these things do not come up – then we will be able to have interactions free of them. But no matter how much we practise, things don't get any better. We have to realize at some point that the way to get better at social interaction is to do it.

There are times when we find ourselves involved in conversations that are ended abruptly. We learn quickly that people can end conversations in a range of ways that go from graceful to extremely hostile.

If the conversation ends when we don't want it to, there is often a feeling of rejection. When that happens, it feels like the walls are closing in on us and all we want to do is escape the situation. But we can force ourselves to deal with it.

❋ We decide to stay, and to "be with our breathing"

❋ We remember that we are not in a threatening situation

Then a miracle happens. Five minutes later we are back to normal. The walls are back where they should be, and we are no longer feeling threatened. That's when a powerful insight hits us: rejection is just a feeling. If it's just a feeling, then we know how to deal with it, in our mindfulness practice. Once we are aware of it, we can tell ourselves: "I am not this feeling, this feeling is not me". Then we recognize that this is true not just of rejection. It's true of other emotions as well: anger, hurt, humiliation are all just feelings too. Suddenly we have something we can practise: we can direct our attention to our emotions and remind ourselves that they are what they are: just feelings.

In a social setting, it may not be possible to take the time out to profoundly contemplate these feelings – we have to explore them in the here and now, with people swirling around us. In a social situation such as a party, the feedback is instant and dynamic; there is no way to control what is happening. We have to be with everything right there in the middle of chaos, without the benefit of time or space. But if, in spite of those challenges, we still allow ourselves to look directly at the emotions assailing us, their power will fade.

When we avoid something, it generally means we are afraid of experiencing it. That fear of feeling a painful emotion controls us. We put a lot of energy into avoiding that painful feeling. But until we have the capacity and courage to just be with these emotions, it is not possible for them to be transformed. When we look at them, acknowledge them and make friends with the feelings we don't like, our fear of experiencing them decreases. They lose their power to control us because when the painful feeling comes up, we no longer try to avoid it.

So, to return to the original question, if practising mindfulness can put us into a state where social interaction is natural and effortless, why can't it transform us so that it will always be that way? It is because when mindfulness is powerful enough, we don't experience rejection and humiliation. And that's the problem. Without being able to experience rejection we cannot come to understand that rejection is just a feeling. Without being able to experience a feeling of humiliation, we cannot transform it.

Generating those feelings with any degree of authenticity whilst sitting on the cushion is rather hard – although it can be done. It is much better to go out and allow it to happen naturally in our interactions with others and to practise with it in that moment. We know from experience that this is extremely difficult – it's easy to shut down and leave. If that happens, go and try it again another day. It's just practice, after all.

Encouraging others in wider society

What really helps most when we are aspiring to help others is our own presence. We won't have any idea what will actually help until we connect with others and have a real sense of what their experiences are. In order to be fully present and connected with another person, we have to be willing to feel whatever comes up in our own experience.

For example, we may be with a friend who is going through a painful personal situation. We might find that, as we sit with them, we begin to feel a lot of intense feelings ourselves. We may feel sadness, anger or bewilderment. We might be sharing our friend's feelings in that moment. Alternatively, we could be experiencing personal reactions to what the person is telling us. Maybe we've been through a similar situation ourselves and perhaps listening to our friend brings up painful feelings of our own. Remember the example we gave, in which someone could not understand how a close friend of theirs could fail to recognize, let alone empathize with, their problems? We need to be aware that what we are feeling and what other people are feeling are not necessarily the same.

Even more commonly, when we want to be helpful, we don't really have a clue what will help. The ability to stay present in the face of uncertainty, unknowing, or even feeling stupid is enormously valuable – despite the fact that it is very hard to do. Sometimes we jump in prematurely with suggestions, stories of our own – or, even worse, with premature snap-judgement advice – just to get away from the discomfort we are feeling ourselves. When we do that, the other person doesn't feel heard or feels put off. They may even shut down and stop talking with us.

The ability to be present without pulling away from discomfort is an important part of mindfulness. It's easy to give yourself the instruction "stay present!" but it's actually quite difficult to do. You'll know this from your own experience, having begun practising by reading and using the exercises in this book. But keep on doing it, continue practising it and you will experience the joy of becoming better and better at it over time.

We can also practise bringing non-judgemental awareness to other kinds of activities such as sports, playing a musical instrument or cooking. In fact, anything that trains us to keep coming back to the present moment without judging what we find will help us become people who can be there for others.

Having compassion does not mean suffering with another person. A quality closely aligned to compassion is gentleness. Gentleness is a way of being kind to ourselves and to others. It means letting go of our tendency to be self-critical, to be aggressive towards ourselves and stand in judgement of ourselves – things that we in the West are so good at. Try instead to work with the question: "is there any way to be gentler with myself (or the other person) about this?"

We can enhance our capacity to be gentle when we do our mindfulness practice. For example, when we realize that we've been caught up in thoughts, we can gently return to the present moment, or to our breath, without adding any extra self-criticism or harshness.

In fact, it is impossible to think of any situations in which mindfulness wouldn't be helpful in some way. Whether it is working with a health issue, negotiating a difficult relationship, parenting a child or making a business deal, knowing what's actually going on in ourselves and the world around us gives us a better chance of relating to the situation wisely.

And this can have a ripple effect – the more people there are who are practising mindfulness, the more the benefits can spread, not just in their own lives, but to the people they live, work and socialize with. The more we see the effect of this on others, the more likely we are to be inspired to practice mindfulness ourselves and to spread the word and the practice. Over time, we might find that the effects of mindfulness – greater awareness, resilience, discernment, compassion – reach enough people that they start to be enjoyed as part of the mainstream of our social fabric. This could become the norm, rather than the exception.

It's important to restate, however, that this process starts with us. We cannot and should not try to force mindfulness onto the world as yet another externally imposed "remedy". That wouldn't be in the gentle spirit of mindfulness and it probably wouldn't work, either.

Hopefully, as we gain a better understanding of the value mindfulness imparts to our everyday life, we will expand our understanding of what mindfulness is – and how it offers us benefits beyond the fields of self-help, benefits that extend into the wider realm of society as a whole.

Mindfulness, by enhancing our self-esteem, helps us to make greater contributions to the community and society that we are living in. Individuals with high levels of self-esteem are happier, perform better and are more aware of the interconnectedness of humans, societies and countries. This awareness can motivate us to make a contribution to others who are less fortunate and to appreciate the gifts of kindness and compassion shown to us by others.

Life is truly an ever-expanding spiral. The more we give, the more we will feel better about ourselves and improve our self-esteem. It is important to note that social change begins with the individual – with ourselves. From the individual it can extend to the immediate family and community, eventually leading to global change.

PART THREE

Mindfulness:
for real

10

Mindfulness for stress, anxiety and depression

Every one of us experiences stress and anxiety at one time or another. Stress is a bodily response to a threat in a situation. Anxiety is a reaction to the stress. But some people experience these feelings uncomfortably often, to a worrying degree, and for no apparent reason, making it difficult for them to carry on with their normal, everyday functioning. These people may have an anxiety disorder, depression or both.

It is not uncommon for someone with an anxiety disorder to also suffer from depression – or vice versa. Nearly one half of those people diagnosed with depression are also diagnosed with having an anxiety disorder. The good news is that these disorders are both treatable. There are various ways to deal with these emotional challenges, but we will be focusing here on mindfulness-based approaches. Before we get to that, we will briefly investigate what stress, anxiety and depression actually mean.

Stress: a common feature in all our lives

When our mind and body perceive a challenge, they release a cascade of hormones to protect and ready themselves. We know this as the "fight or flight" response. Beta-endorphins (along with epinephrine and norepinephrine) are the hormones that kick in to produce it: they are responsible for decreasing our ability to feel pain and yet leaving us capable of undertaking remarkable acts of courage. Once the emergency is over, the body returns to a more relaxed state.

Prostaglandin is one member of this pack of hormones that you might not be familiar with. But it is highly significant: it tells our immune system to ready itself for attack. Serotonin is a bit better known, being notorious for its role in antidepressants: it is an important chemical messenger in relaying communications in the nervous system. If your serotonin levels are high, you're happy.

Adrenalin is probably the best known of all. It provides a natural high and is the reason why we enjoy extreme sports and action movies, as the frisson of danger and excitement they produce is geared towards releasing it. Many of us might find ourselves seeking out ever more challenging pastimes, situations and activities in order to feel the effects of adrenalin, as a state of stress is all too often our default mode in our high-pressure modern lives.

Cortisol is the main hormone secreted from the adrenal glands, which lie near the kidneys. Its main function is to provide resistance to a variety of stresses and maintain the activity of a variety of enzyme systems. All of this requires energy, which is supplied by the liver, releasing increasing amounts of glucose into our blood.

So that's how it all works. But what can we do about these stress reactions? Let's go back to the top of the chain: the brain. We can make decisions that help eliminate or decrease the stress response in our life by becoming more sensitive to the physical and emotional components of our health.

We suffer from a multitude of **physical stressors** (phenomena that cause stress). They might include such things as physical accidents, changes in temperature and even inactivity. (Yes, although it might not seem like it, inactivity can itself up our stress levels.) **Chemical stressors** include sugar, high-fat foods, cigarettes and alcohol. Our workplaces and even our homes might be breeding grounds of chemical stressors – a computer printer perched on the end of your desk, or traffic fumes coming into your apartment. **Emotional stressors** include fear, anger, guilt, depression, anxiety and loneliness.

Many of us work our stress capacity to overload. If we have a difficult family get-together to navigate, we might perhaps start eating poorly, or abruptly stop our regular exercise regimen. But it is possible to come up with a plan for how we can minimize the effect of these stressors by planning ahead.

Make sure you are able to identify when your stress levels are high and identify some ways to interrupt the process. An increased heart-rate, tense muscles, irritability, moodiness, breaking out into a sweat, clamminess, and dilated pupils are all clear signs of the "fight or flight" mechanism kicking in: a heightened stress response. When you notice these signs, you should stop what you're doing and check in with yourself for a few moments. There are many ways to reset the system. These might include:

* going for a brisk walk
* visualizing yourself somewhere refreshing
* relaxing any tight muscles and shifting your perception to a completely different space

✳ indulging yourself in the three-minute breathing space exercise (see p.74)

Resetting yourself every couple of hours or so with the three-minute exercise is bound to ultimately make you feel some shift in your overall tension pattern. But use whatever works for you.

Sometimes, however, our stress patterns are so deeply ingrained that we are unable to recognize, identify or change them on our own. If you decide that this is the case, it might be a good time to seek the help of a professional. We might now also remember what we have read so far about mindfulness and draw some conclusions about the value of this way of being to address stress in our lives. So if you have been reading this book but have not started practising mindfulness yet, then perhaps now you should turn to Part 2 and start putting mindfulness into action.

We mainly see stress as a negative emotion

The hormonal cascade described above is a healthy and natural response to a hard (or potentially dangerous) situation. Problems occur when our system does not reset itself. Chronic stress – when your body doesn't go back to resting, when the chemicals inside us don't go back to their baseline levels – can alter our health and activate disease. We all react to stress and cope with it in different ways: it is these differences that determine whether or not stress becomes a negative force in our life.

Stress is essentially an imbalance between the demands placed on us and our ability to cope with those demands. Pressure can come from a variety of sources – it might be moving house, money worries or relationship problems. But most frequently, work is the biggest stressor. According to the Samaritans (a UK charity that offers emotional support for those in distress), one in five people suffer from unmanageable stress on a daily basis, and the Health and Safety Executive in the UK reports that one in three instances of all work-related illness are due to stress.

Anxiety

Although we may not realize it, anxiety is with us all, at varying levels of intensity, throughout our lives. Everybody has anxiety. It is a part of being alive – part of our natural, in-built survival kit. When crossing a busy street, we may be anxious, deep down, about being run over by a car: without anxiety we wouldn't be careful when we crossed the road. There is an extent to which a fear of failure, or of humiliation, produces an anxiety without which our performance in public situations simply would be nowhere near as good. This is as true for athletes and entertainers as it is for business executives giving a presentation, or students taking an exam.

> *To have anxiety is to be human.*

Mild threat or danger makes us nervous and slightly anxious. But in times of real danger, anxiety comes upon us swiftly and is much stronger: we need to take action urgently. When the threat is imminent, it turns to panic and brings with it all panic's symptoms: a racing heart, fast breathing, trembling, breaking into a sweat and the like. These come on almost instantly. That's just how anxiety works.

Problems with anxiety arise when we start to feel anxious more often and more intensely than any challenges or danger require; when anxiety occurs seemingly without reason. It is this persistent, unexplained anxiety that can give rise to a whole host of related problems and disorders.

Depression

Depression is a condition in which we feel discouraged, sad, hopeless, unmotivated or disinterested in life in general. We are probably all guilty of over-using the word "depressed" in everyday life. Sometimes we say "I'm depressed" when in fact what we really mean is "I'm fed up". We might have had an argument with a friend, or failed a test or lost out on a job promotion. These ups and downs in life are normal and commonplace. When these feelings last for a short period of time, it may just be a case of "the blues" – feeling a little bit down. Most of us recover quite quickly.

In a case of more serious depression, however, the sufferer will experience a low mood and other symptoms every day for two weeks or more. Symptoms can become severe enough to utterly undermine our normal day-to-day activities. This might be the point at which a diagnosis of clinical depression is made. Such intense and protracted symptoms can be devastating: so profoundly unbearable that a sufferer may contemplate ending their life.

The UK's National Health Service asserts that around two in three of us have depression at some point in our life. Sometimes it is mild, lasting just a few weeks. However, an episode of depression serious enough to require treatment occurs among more people than you would think: about one in four women and one in ten men are diagnosed as being depressed at some point in their lives. Among those people, many will experience a relapse and will go on to further episodes at various times in their life.

Depression is common, but many people don't admit that they have experienced it. Some feel there is a stigma attached or that people will think them weak if they admit it. Yet great leaders such as Winston Churchill have suffered from depression: he was described by his political colleague and friend Lord Beaverbrook as always either "at the top of the wheel of confidence or at the bottom of an intense depression". Depression is one of the most common illnesses that doctors deal with. People with depression may be unhelpfully told by others to "pull their socks up" or "snap out of it". The truth is, they cannot, and such comments by others are very unhelpful. Even worse, they may bottle up their symptoms to hide them from friends and relatives. But, if they are encouraged to be open about their feelings with close family and friends, it may help them to be understood.

Some people are afraid that they are going mad. Understanding that the symptoms they are experiencing may be indicative of depression, and that they are far from unique in this, may help sufferers to accept that they are ill and need professional help. When such feelings last for more than two weeks without pause, and when the feelings interfere with daily activities such as taking care of family, spending time with friends or going to work or school, it is likely that the person is experiencing an episode of clinical depression.

One approach to enable people to learn how to deal with stress, anxiety and depression is mindfulness. There are several established paths towards mindfulness, sometimes described as Mindfulness-based Applications (MBA) or Mindfulness-based Interventions (MBI).

MBAs, MBIs and other paths to mindfulness

Mindfulness-based approaches are training programmes, usually delivered over an eight-week period, that are intended to teach people practical mindfulness skills in a step-by-step process. These enable participants to cope differently with physical and psychological health problems, as well as ongoing life challenges.

Over time, a variety of mindfulness-based approaches have been developed for different target groups and situations. The most common are:

* Mindfulness-based Stress Reduction Programme (MBSR)
* Mindfulness-based Cognitive Therapy (MBCT)
* MBCT for Chronic Fatigue Syndrome
* MBCT for Cancer Patients
* Mindfulness-based Relapse Prevention (MBRP) for Addictive Trappings of the Mind
* Mindfulness-based Mind Fitness Training (MMFT) for Military Personnel
* Mindfulness-based Approaches to Eating Disorders
* MBSR for Urban Youth
* MBCT for Anxious Children
* Mindfulness for Schools
* Mindfulness at Work
* MbM-Management by Meditation™
* Mindfulness-based Awareness Coaching (MBAC) for Individuals and Organizations

We'll now take a closer look at the two main approaches: the Mindfulness-based Stress Reduction Programme (MBSR) and Mindfulness-based Cognitive Therapy (MBCT), both of which are training programmes that are usually delivered in eight weekly sessions of between two and three and a half hours in length.

Mindfulness-based Stress Reduction (MBSR)

Jon Kabat-Zinn developed MBSR – the first mindfulness-based training course – at the University of Massachusetts Medical Centre in 1979. It was initially designed to work with, and provide relief for, patients experiencing chronic and intractable physical pain. MBSR is the foundation of all of the mindfulness programmes that have been developed subsequently and is now offered in over two hundred medical centres, hospitals and clinics around the world.

Since its inception, MBSR has evolved into a common form of complementary medicine addressing a variety of health problems. The National Institutes of Health's National Center for Complementary and Alternative Medicine in the US provided a number of grants to research the efficacy of the MBSR programme in promoting healing. Many universities, research institutes and researchers followed and over the last 34 years a large number of scientific papers have substantiated the efficacy of MBSR. Amongst the findings from this wealth of research are that pain-related drug utilization can be decreased and that activity levels and feelings of self-esteem increased for a majority of participants. Whilst the healing element of MBSR is the most significant, there is also the aspect of prevention and wellness. It is about learning how to take good care of yourself and how to achieve a greater sense of balance through health enhancement.

Mindfulness practice allows us to cultivate a greater awareness of the unity of mind and body, as well as helping to reveal the ways unconscious thoughts, feelings and behaviours can undermine physical and mental health. The MBSR programme brings meditation and mindful yoga together so that the virtues of both can be experienced simultaneously.

Many of the MBSR programmes are taught by physicians, nurses, social workers and psychologists, as well as other health professionals and, more recently, school teachers and business coaches. They are seeking to reclaim and deepen some of the reciprocity inherent in the relationships between, say:

* Health practitioner and patient
* Teacher and student
* Coach and coachee

This approach is founded in an active, participatory partnership; a partnership in which the patient, student or coachee takes on significant responsibility for doing a specific kind of interior work to enable them to tap into their own deepest inner resources for learning, growing, healing and transformation.

How does MBSR help?

Stress, in MBSR, is symptomatic of "general suffering". In the MBSR classroom we work with our body, with our breath and with our mind to reduce our suffering regardless of the source or stressor. MBSR is a unique programme that challenges us to reduce the impact of the stress we experience in our lives – not by eliminating the things that stress us out, but by changing how we relate to them.

As human beings we have a lot in common:
We all have a body
We all have a mind
We all are breathing
And we all are suffering.
Jon Kabat-Zinn

In this frenetic world, large numbers of us experience tension, sleeplessness and physical discomfort from stress. Left unrelieved, stress not only eats away at our happiness, but is destructive to our health in many ways. In the box opposite are listed some signs of excessive stress: we call them stress indicators.

What if we could reduce the impact of stress – even if our outer circumstances didn't change? This is precisely what MBSR seeks to achieve. MBSR is best described as "meditative awareness". It helps those practising it to "enter into a new relationship with chronic pain, anxiety and depression." So what does that mean? Well, by being trained in MBSR, we learn how to better observe experiences, instead of being completely immersed in them. This impartial stance is often described as the "witness state" – the ability to simply observe what we are thinking and feeling at the very same time that we are having those thoughts and feelings. MBSR helps us to strengthen that "witnessing" aspect of ourselves, providing a constant, always-present tool to use in situations of pain, anxiety or stress.

Picture your thoughts as though they were a stream. Most of the time, we are right in the middle of the swirling water, but we can make a conscious decision to go over to the bank and stand there, watching the water flowing by. We may step into the water, consciously, or we may become aware we are in it already, but we can also consciously decide to return to the bank. With practice, we will have something solid to stand on as our emotions and sensations are flowing by.

Similarly, when we are in an angry state, feeling the urge to engage in an aggressive action, the initial impulse will pass away quickly if we can be mindful of it, if we can simply be with the discomfort and wait for it to go. Once that has happened, we are in a position to make real choices about our behaviour.

A list of common stress indicators

Physiological reactions
Blood pressure increases
Heart rate increases
Increased blood flow to
  muscles
Increase in stress hormones
Immune system changes
Perspiration increases

Behavioural reactions
Biting nails
Clenching/grinding teeth
Finger/toe tapping
Procrastination
Social withdrawal
Critical attitude towards
  others
Compulsive eating
Drug and alcohol abuse

Emotional reactions
Worry/anxiety
Irritability/short fuse
Intense emotions
  (fear, anger, distress)
Boredom/withdrawal
Loss of pleasure
Decreased sense of humour

Cognitive reactions
Racing thoughts
Obsessive thinking
Decreased concentration
Indecisiveness
Lack of creativity

Physical reactions
Increased muscle tension
Headache
Increased pain
Sleep problems
Fatigue or restlessness
Digestive problems

We often observe the moment when our participants actually get this concept, through ongoing practice. It is not something which comes from a book or a particular lecture – it is the practice of mindfulness that takes them to it.

What's involved in MBSR sessions?

Each MBSR session typically consists of

✳ **The topic of the week**

❋ Time for mindfulness practice

❋ Enquiry, to reflect upon the participant's experience of meditating and living mindfully

❋ Reflection on the homework

❋ Preparation for the next training step and the homework for the week ahead

Participants are usually provided with recordings to support their practice at home – which will involve the body scan, mindful yoga and a sitting practice. The yoga practice can be modified to accommodate most participants, even those who have an illness or chronic pain that limits their movement. In these eight consecutive weeks the following should be covered:

❋ Recognizing the present moment

❋ Perception and creative responding

❋ The pleasure and power in being present

❋ Stress reactivity

❋ Stress response

❋ Mindful communication

❋ Integrating mindfulness into daily life

❋ How to keep up the momentum

MBSR is designed to help us feel well, regardless of what is going on, even if we are filled with anxiety or pain. We can learn how to experience wellbeing despite the situation we find ourselves in. It is not just about having a quiet mind. It is a practice we can take into our busy daily life.

Homework activities, designed to strengthen practice, are generally assigned to participants so that mindfulness becomes a habit and consequently a skill that is applicable in any situation. We recommend that those who are interested in such a programme consider enrolling for MBSR when they are able to attend all sessions, to ensure the greatest success.

Mindfulness One-Day Retreat

One key element of mindfulness practice is the one-day retreat between session six and seven. In this day we create the space to practise, we experience practising mindfulness as a group as well as on our own, because it is a day of silence. This means that even whilst we are in a group of meditators, we stay with ourselves; we don't interact with each other.

During this day we are able to deepen our mindfulness practice and enhance our mindfulness skills. We investigate our personal relationship to the breath, body, feelings and thoughts while we are sitting, standing, lying or walking.

Throughout this day, we are engaged in an internal journey and will experience a range of "weather conditions". There may be stormy thoughts and emotions which lead us away from being in the here and now. There might be also darker moments when we ask ourselves "what on earth am I doing here?". There will also be those moments when the sun breaks through the dark clouds and lights up the mind, bringing us back to the awareness of the present moment and to a stress-free encounter with ourselves.

Not having experienced it, some may feel a little apprehensive about spending a long time in silence, practising meditation. However, almost everyone reports feeling deeply refreshed and restored by this day. They find that the practice gets embodied in a way that they have not experienced by having only done shorter practices in the group or at home.

What do we learn in MBSR?

More than three decades of published research indicate that the majority of people who complete an MBSR programme report:

* an increased ability to relax

* greater energy and enthusiasm for life

* an ability to cope more effectively with both short and long-term stressful situations

* major improvement in pain-related anxiety, depression, hostility and the tendency to become preoccupied with painful sensations in both body and mind

* lasting decreases in difficult physical and psychological symptoms

* reductions in pain levels, with an enhanced ability to cope with pain that may not go way

Mindfulness-Based Cognitive Therapy (MBCT)

Based on the "mother programme" (MBSR), Dr Zindel Segal (Toronto), Dr Mark Williams (Oxford) and Dr John Teasdale (Cambridge) developed Mindfulness-Based Cognitive Therapy (MBCT) by implementing relevant aspects of cognitive behavioural therapy (CBT) into mindfulness.

MBCT was primarily developed to help people suffering from depression. Research evidence has confirmed its efficacy in preventing relapses in recurrently depressed participants who have made a recovery, through teaching them skills to disengage from habitual "automatic" unhelpful cognitive patterns. MBCT has been shown to halve the relapse rate in recovered patients with three or more episodes of depression. It is effective in preventing "autonomous" relapses but not those provoked by stressful events. Since 2009 the UK's National Health Service (NHS) via the National Institute for Clinical Excellence (NICE) has promoted the use of MBCT in dealing with relapsing depression, thereby highlighting the possibilities of mindfulness in general and mindfulness in combination with cognitive behaviour therapy.

As outlined previously, the pattern of mind which makes people vulnerable to depressive relapse is rumination, in which the mind repetitively reruns negative thoughts. The core skill that MBCT teaches is to intentionally "shift mental gears". MBCT differs from conventional CBT in that it does not place an emphasis on changing the content of thoughts. The focus in MBCT is on a systematic training to be more aware, moment by moment of physical sensations, feelings and thoughts. This facilitates a "decentred" relationship to body sensations, feelings and thoughts from which they can then be seen as aspects of experience which move through our awareness and which are not necessarily reality in any given moment.

What is the core of MBCT?

The MBCT programme takes place over eight weeks with a two-hour session each week. However, the main work is done at home between the sessions. A set of recordings are provided to accompany the programme, and these are used by participants to practise at home for six out of seven days. The session structure itself is very similar to that of the MBSR programme. During the sessions, opportunities are provided to talk about participants' experiences with their home practices, the obstacles that inevitably arise and how to deal with them skilfully.

The specific themes addressed in the MBCT programme are:

* Session 1: automatic pilot
* Session 2: dealing with barriers
* Session 3: mindfulness of the breath
* Session 4: staying present
* Session 5: allowing and letting be

❋ Session 6: thoughts are not facts

❋ Session 7: how can I best take care of myself?

❋ Session 8: using what's been learned to deal with future moods

Over the eight weeks of the programme, the mindfulness practices taught in the sessions help participants to become more familiar with the workings of the mind. MBCT allows us to notice the times when we are at risk of getting caught in old habitual patterns of mind that re-activate downward spirals in mood. It allows us to explore ways of releasing ourselves from those old habits and – if we choose – enter a different way of being.

How will MBCT help us to prevent depression relapse?

In the very first place, MBCT helps us to understand what depression is. From this deeper understanding, we are able to go on to discover what makes us vulnerable to downward spirals in mood and why we get stuck at the bottom of the spiral.

Once we know how we travel into the danger zone, we can start to explore how we spring the trap on ourselves. Often we feel pushed to meet impossibly high standards set by ourselves or others and we may be left feeling that we are "not good enough" if we are not able to meet them. There is a whole host of ways in which we put ourselves under pressure, or we may be placed under pressure by others. Work overload may make us miserable and there is a myriad of other issues which may mean that we lose touch with what makes life worth living.

The discovery that, even when we feel well, the link between negative moods and negative thoughts remains ready to be reactivated, is of enormous importance. It means that sustaining recovery from such depression depends on learning how to keep mild states of depression from spiralling out of control.

Which programme fits me best?

This is a question that this book cannot answer conclusively. If you have become curious and are considering whether a mindfulness eight-week training programme would be beneficial to you, you should look for a competent provider of these programmes and ask for an individual consultation. There you will find your answer. In Chapter 14 we will suggest tested and proven resources and providers for you to continue your journey with.

However, it is quite possible that neither MBSR nor MBCT may be suitable for the issues you face, or an appropriate choice for you at this time. This may be the case if you are dealing with:

* Substance abuse or dependence (currently or within the past year)
* An acute medical problem requiring frequent intervention or treatment
* Psychological issues such as trauma, severe depression, psychosis, active suicidal thoughts (or other major psychiatric diagnosis)

We must make it clear that neither MBSR nor MBCT are psychotherapeutic interventions. These programmes are *not* a substitute for mental health therapy or counselling, for medical care or for substance abuse treatment.

In addition, it might be useful to keep in mind that the eight-week programmes always contain gentle stretching and yoga exercises. Although very gentle, they may be beyond some people's capabilities and, as with all exercise programmes, if you are not sure if they are suitable for you, you should consult a professional medical practitioner. In general we would recommend that you work with somebody who knows what he or she is doing. There are many well-trained MBSR or MBCT teachers out there – teachers who are practising on a daily basis for themselves. We call this "walking the talk"; this is a real quality mark and the most important requirement in all "Best Practice Guidelines" for MBA teachers and MBA teacher trainers (see resources in Chapter 14).

Key differences between MBSR and MBCT

Although the two programmes are broadly similar and are often used flexibly, the key ways in which MBCT differs from MBSR are as follows.

MBCT tends to target specific conditions or vulnerabilities, whereas MBSR has a more generic application – it is applied to stress that arises from a variety of life events including physical or mental illness. Both MBSR and MBCT bring about psychological insights concerning our experiences and difficulties and aim to develop skills to deal with these differently. MBCT puts a greater emphasis on working with, and understanding, the psychological and cognitive aspects of our experience.

Both MBSR and MBCT integrate the dynamic, "in-the-moment responding" aspect of mindfulness, with an understanding of the origins and maintenance factors of the unhelpful behaviours or psychopathology being dealt with. Both MBSR and MBCT draw on concepts and skills from other disciplines. For example, MBSR includes teaching on everyday communication and lifestyle, while MBCT includes techniques and exercises from cognitive behavioural therapy and includes didactic elements, which give the participants information about a particular difficulty. In the case of depression, for instance, participants are given information on the *universal* characteristics of depression, to help them recognize and deal with the signatures of their relapses.

11

Mindfulness and work

Employers know that decision-making skills, creativity, problem-solving skills, focus and concentration are all compromised by prolonged and ongoing stress. Work-related stress caused workers in the UK to lose 10.8 million working days between 2010 and 2011. On average, each person suffering from this condition took 27 days off work, according to the Health and Safety Executive.

The American Psychological Association reports that:

* Forty-eight percent of the American workforce felt that stress was having a negative impact on their personal and professional life

* Thirty-one percent of employed adults said that they had difficulty managing work and family responsibilities

* Thirty-five percent claimed that their job's interference with their family or personal time was a significant source of stress

* Fifty-four percent said stress had caused them to fight with people close to them

✱ Twenty-six percent reported being alienated from a
friend or family member because of stress

The annual costs to employers in stress-related health care
and missed work amounted to $300 billion in 2011 with thirty
percent of employees claiming they are "always" or "often"
under stress at work.

The mindful workplace: innovation and productivity

Research into the effects of mindfulness meditation programmes and the experience of an increasing number of
corporations all over the world confirm that mindfulness
meditation gets positive results; human resourcefulness and
creativity is activated and enhanced when in a state of inner
calm and relaxation. Memory improves, as does the ability to
envision different options, shift perspective, see opportunities,
collaborate and discover solutions.

According to the National Institutes of Health, the University of Massachusetts and the Mind and Body Medical Institute at Harvard University, mindfulness enhances the qualities
companies need most from their workforce:

✱ increased brain-wave activity

✱ enhanced intuition

✱ better concentration

✱ alleviation of the aches and pains that plague
employees most

Organizations are now recognizing the value of workplace mindfulness programmes to generate positive results
in executive performance, employee engagement, employee
retention, customer service and bottom-line results.

Dr Britta Hölzel, a research fellow at MGH and Giessen University in Germany found, that by practising mindfulness meditation, we can play an active role in changing the brain. Hölzel's research indicates that mindfulness training in the workplace results in:

* improved self-esteem
* increased coping and stress management skills
* an enhanced ability to relax and enjoy life
* improved energy and a greater sense of happiness
* improved work-related performance
* enhanced ability to respond (rather than react) to situations, improved concentration and mental focus
* enhanced self-management skills

Mindfulness and business schools

Business schools too are beginning to embrace this practice. The teaching and studying of mindfulness has become very popular in the corporate world.

Master of Business Administration (MBA) and executive education courses are two of the most significant and popular career-enhancing pieces of training in the business world, and there are now lecturers in both who offer mindfulness-based techniques to help students calm their minds and increase their focus. Such skills, they argue, are crucial for those hoping to succeed in an increasingly frenetic environment where there are a range of burdens: from the distractions of an always-ringing phone to pressure for strong quarterly profits. That instantaneous decisions are made about matters with potentially serious consequences is usually just part of the job.

While the idea of mindfulness – as we now know – originates in the daily practice of meditation, business school faculties see it as having many applications for executives who aren't looking for a spiritual dimension but simply want to clear their heads and become aware of reflexive, emotional reactions that can lead to bad decisions.

According to a report from INSEAD (a leading European business school based in France), coaching based on introspection and meditative techniques, as well as mindfulness-based leadership interventions, resulted in behaviours that were more likely to lead to greater levels of Corporate Social Responsibility (CSR). A total of 427 interviews were conducted in 19 companies across 8 different corporate sectors. This included a one-day in-depth fact-finding mission, with eleven interviews with senior executives and CSR managers.

We can confirm from our own work – coaching executives and offering support for organizational development – that organizations that have adopted mindfulness techniques tend to pay close attention to what is happening within them. They are ready to correct mistakes rather than punishing workers who report them and respond quickly to changes and/or problems.

As reported by *The Wall Street Journal*, Donde Ashmos Plowman, dean of the University of Nebraska-Lincoln College of Business Administration, decided to conduct some research into how mindful other business schools were in the US – in terms of such simple acts as noticing new things and being aware of their own workings. She sent out a questionnaire to deans and other administrators of 180 business schools.

She had been prompted by the accusation of critics that the attitudes of business schools were partly responsible for the many high-profile lapses of corporate ethics in recent years. Plowman was trying to find out just how mindful these institutions were in their attitudes: how focused and self-aware they were about what happened in them. She was interested in establishing how – or indeed whether – they were capable of self-correction.

Perhaps the most interesting of her findings was that the deans of these schools – the people at the top – consistently rated their schools' self-awareness more highly than did those working for them. "It's easy for people at the head of an organization to end up in a bubble", she said. "That really alerted me to say, 'What do I need to do as a dean to improve the way we communicate?'" So what *do* they need to do to improve the way they communicate?

The ones that actually do a good job

Leadership professor Ben Bryant works at the IMD Business School in Lausanne, Switzerland. He introduces his executive-education students to techniques for concentrating on their breathing; he wants them to become aware of sounds and sensations, to help them centre themselves – whether they are in the office, at their desk or in a business meeting.

Whilst it is true, as many proponents of meditation would assert, that the practice was never meant to be instrumental in making money, it must surely be worthwhile to help those running companies to slow down and think about how best to direct their attention.

This is particularly true for those in positions of leadership, the effect of whose smallest decisions may ripple outwards – for good or ill. Because their lives are often frantic and over-burdened, they miss too many opportunities to make either themselves or their organizations different.

Jeremy Hunter, recently appointed Professor of Practice at the Peter Drucker School of Management, Claremont

Graduate School in California, believes mindfulness should be at the centre of business schools' teaching. That, he argues, is because it is about improving the quality of attention. In the modern workplace, attention is the key to productivity. In a series of four seven-week executive-education classes and a separate course for MBA students, Professor Hunter teaches what he calls "self-management". He often starts class with a brief meditation and covers topics such as managing emotional reactions and dealing with change.

One of the key advantages of mindful approaches being available at business schools is that they are able to reach a sceptical audience that would never normally attend a meditation class. By encountering the practices in a business context, participants are given the opportunity to recognize the techniques' usefulness. In one discussion about multi-tasking, a student raised his frustration with a weekly work meeting in which members of staff were more focused on their mobile phones, iPads and BlackBerries than on the discussion. On Professor Hunter's advice he returned to the office and insisted that everyone put their phones in a box before starting. Colleagues initially responded with irritation, but the weekly gathering soon became so much more efficient that it was cut down from ninety minutes to an hour.

At Harvard Business School, Professor William George focuses on helping people in business to better understand their emotions. He has meditated regularly since 1975 and in 2010 ran a two-day conference on mindful leadership with a Tibetan Buddhist meditation master.

Without a powerful sense of self-awareness, Professor George feels leaders often have difficulty acknowledging mistakes and will be more likely to fall prey to the temptations of power and money that their position gives them access to. On the other hand, MBA degree candidates who learn the discipline of mindfulness tend to become more understanding and more motivational as leaders.

Organizations which now offer mindfulness training to their staff include: Astra Zeneca, AXA PPP, Deutsche Bank, eBay, GlaxoSmithKline, KPMG, Google, Apple, the NHS, the Cabinet Office, The Home Office, the military (in both the UK and US), Procter and Gamble, Starbucks, Skype and Yahoo, to name but a few. That list ought to make it clear that mindfulness is certainly no longer a fringe activity.

The mindful leader

If organizations were mindful leadership would be quite a different matter. Whilst autocratic leadership is no longer a real option for those who wish to be truly effective as leaders, simply being mindful on their own account is not sufficient either. Without promoting mindfulness throughout the whole organization and across the whole workforce, they would be failing in their most important responsibility – enabling their employees to be mindful as well and bringing about a shift in their organization's culture.

Noticing what is around us puts us in the present, makes us sensitive to context and aware of change and uncertainty. When we are mindless, our perspective is at a standstill. We fall into the trap of confusing the stasis of our mindset with the stability of the underlying phenomena. However visionary we consider our leaders, they cannot predict the future any more than anyone else. They may be able to predict what might happen – if they're good at their job, they might even be able to do this most of the time, if situations stay constant but they can never accurately forecast all events. Even when repeating something which has had an identical outcome on each previous occasion, there is no guarantee that the next time we do the same thing the same outcome will follow.

Those in positions of power often keep quiet about what they don't know. When they do confess to not knowing something, they generally do so defensively. They work from the assumption: "I don't know, but it is nonetheless knowable and I probably should know." True leaders should stand up for uncertainty: "I don't know, and you don't know, because it is unknowable." When leaders acknowledge this universal truth, they can be less distracted by the need to appear to be all-knowing, allowing them to get on with the real problems at hand. Being awake in the moment allows us all to better understand what we all need to know just right now.

The best companies have leaders with a vision. A vision gives a direction even when we cannot be certain that we will reach our goals. But to create a vision, leaders need to know what is really important and what impact it might have. They need authenticity rather than bureaucratic authority. Real charisma is hard-won: it is born out of empathy, integrity and compassion. These are the kind of leadership competences built by mindfulness!

How we see our colleagues and staff

Mindlessness can lead us to assumptions about behaviour. But when we understand the other's perspective, we can be less judgemental; and when we do we'll find we have a less inflexible view of people. For example, if we perceive someone as being rigid, we will ignore them and their point of view. If, however, we see them as consistent, as someone who can be counted on, we will value them.

We can turn around every judgement in this way; so rather

than seeing someone as impulsive, perceive them as spontaneous, rather than grim as serious, and rather than eager to please, see them as seeking harmony. Once we free ourselves from our misplaced superiority, we may find talent and ability in those we had previously denounced.

Even more significantly, if everyone is wide awake, we will no longer need to lead as though everyone needs to be directed or commanded all the time. We may find that people are able to see for themselves what the situation demands, and work towards a common vision. We might find that they can contribute valuable insights and make constructive proposals once they are included, listened to and heard. And the surprising result may be a greatly enhanced performance.

Making beautiful music together

In a study conducted by Ellen Langer, a professor of psychology at Harvard University, orchestral musicians were given playing instructions in which they were directed to be either mindless or mindful. In this case, being mindless meant replicating a previous performance with which they were very satisfied. Being mindful, on the other hand, directed them to make the piece new, albeit in very subtle ways that only they would know. Since they were playing classical music – following the notes on a composed score – the differences were indeed subtle.

Their performance was recorded and then played for audiences unaware of the musicians having been given instructions. The researchers found that not only did the musicians much prefer the experience of playing mindfully, but the mindfully played pieces were judged as superior by the audience. Everyone was, in a sense, mindfully doing their own thing. The result was a better coordinated outcome.

After more than thirty years of research we have sound evidence that practising mindfulness will tend to increase productivity and personal charisma, decrease burnout and the amount of accidents and mistakes, and improve creativity, memory, attention. It has positive effects on health and even longevity. When we are mindful we can take advantage of opportunities and anticipate dangers that don't yet exist. This is true for both the leader and the led.

The illusion of omniscience

There is no "best way" to do anything independent of context. Seen from this perspective, the person in charge never really has privileged information. When leaders seek to keep everyone in their place with the illusion of being all-knowing and in possession of privileged knowledge, they may feel superior, but the price of this is that they create slavish followers instead of an involved workforce. Their mindlessness promotes our own mindlessness which costs us our wellbeing and health. The final result: the leader, the led and the company all lose.

A company in which *everyone* is mindful, with mindful coaches creating a mindful coaching culture, based on a mindful communication culture would be a truly productive, co-operative one. It may take some time to achieve this ideal and to realize this vision. But, in the meantime, we need mindful leaders and mindfulness ambassadors at all levels who understand the urgency of promoting mindfulness in those around them. The mindful movement has started; let's keep it rolling!

Exercise: the STOP exercise

To become part of this movement, a good suggestion to start with might be the STOP exercise. The STOP exercise only needs a few moments: it's a small investment with a huge outcome.

When you practice the STOP exercise, you remain motionless for this moment of observation. You attempt to note your physical position and sensations, emotional states and any thoughts occurring. Notice them, but be aware that you don't start to identify with them.

* **S stands for stop and pause**
  Step out of your "automatic pilot": mode

* **T stands for take a breath (take a moment)**
  Be only with your breathing

* **O stands for observing**

  Observe your physical state. Are you aware of the sensations of your body? Are you in a position of stable balance or an awkward, off-balance position? Are you sensing anything (e.g. touching, tasting, smelling, hearing, seeing)?

  Observe your emotional state. Are you aware of your emotions? Are you worried, angry, depressed or happy?

  Observe your mind state. Are thoughts present? Are you thinking about the past or future? Are you trying to solve problems or improve a situation?

* **P stands for proceed with your agenda**

  Return to your daily routine

We love this practice because it is accessible and practical and doesn't need any special time to be set aside for it. It can be used in so many aspects of life. We might be a frantic parent feeling suddenly overwhelmed by the demands of our child. We might be struggling to cope with the needs of a sick friend or relative. We might be about to lash out in anger, in an escalating argument. Practising STOP for just a moment will help everyone to regain some equilibrium.

You might not work in an office...

You could be a full-time mother, a farmer, a shopkeeper or a cleaner. You may have an occupation that mainly involves physical labour. No matter what your occupation, you can practise mindfulness to build self-esteem all day long! See each task of your working day as a brilliant opportunity to boost your self-esteem. Don't think about what you need to do next. Think about who you are and what you are doing here and now. Be present in yourself and in your movements. After all, you are your most important self-esteem coach: you are the one who creates your own future.

A tool for organizational change

When we discuss Corporate Social Responsibility (CSR), it is almost always contextualized in terms of actions and decision-making at the corporate, structural level. However, at the heart of every corporate practice that touches upon an environmental or social issue, there are *individuals* who are weighing the costs and benefits of taking social responsibility factors into consideration. In our professional capacity at London Meditation we work on mindfulness in the workplace as a tool for change: on an individual, team and organizational level. Whilst we are addressing dysfunction at the micro level – for example in terms of personal discontent, frustration or anger – the impact of this is to effect positive change further up the chain. We see this growing collective consciousness as reflecting the interconnectedness of the natural world – we are all part of a larger, inseparable, organic system.

How does CSR fit in?

By creating greater consciousness at the individual level, we become more mindful of how our actions impact on others, and ultimately, the world around us.

Organizations operate at different levels: the individual, the team, the company itself, the markets in which the company operates, the society in which those markets function and the environment surrounding the company.

But patterns that exist on one single level tend to be replicated across the whole. If we are able to translate the changed patterns we bring about at an individual level we can make this change permeate throughout all the various layers. This leads us to consideration of corporate social responsibility, which focuses on the ethical repercussions of the interaction between these layers.

Changing thought at an individual level

By integrating more holistic environmental, social and governance considerations into the strategy and operations of business, new opportunities emerge – opportunities to reduce failures that cost both business and society. With better organizational structure and increased emphasis on personal and team mindfulness, businesses can become more dynamic and adaptable.

In terms of social responsibility, the time has come to consider how corporate attention can be shifted from purely compliance-based practices to a fundamental rethink aimed at truly addressing human, social and environmental needs. It is perhaps of little surprise that the fundamental qualities of this need were grasped intuitively by remarkable individuals such as Gandhi and Einstein many decades ago. Gandhi put

12 moments to reduce stress at work – a mindful agenda for busy people

1. Start with your formal practice in the morning (the body scan, mindful yoga, or a breathing exercise).

2. If you drive a car, before you turn on the ignition, take a few moments for breath awareness.

3. Whether in a car, cycling or on public transport don't keep your mind turned off (via music, news or audio books). Stay consciously with the experience of driving, or cycling, or the motion of travelling and what it releases inside you.

4. When stopping at the traffic lights or using public transport become aware of your surroundings.

5. Allow yourself to get consciously in touch with your work space when you arrive at your workplace.

6. Pause for one moment and breathe consciously before you open an incoming email or answer a phone call.

7. Remember to relax when you take a break, instead of seeing it only as transfer time from one work sequence to the next.

in the form of this instruction: "Become the change that you wish to see in the world". Albert Einstein once remarked, less poetically but very clearly, that "a man's value to the community depends primarily on how far his feelings, thoughts and actions, are directed to promoting the good of his fellows." He also wrote, in 1950, something that has a more direct application to the worlds of business and companies: "the aim of education must be the training of independently acting and

8. Do only one thing at a time: eating, or reading, or browsing the Internet and if at all possible, change your location at break time.

9. Whenever you become aware that you feel stress, pressure, fear, fatigue, that the pace is too hectic or even that you are bored, then check in: If possible, close your eyes on an in-breath and for a moment turn inward and then open your eyes on an out-breath again.

10. At the end of your working day, consciously complete your last bit of work, say farewell and allow yourself to become aware of the transition from work to leisure time or to going home.

11. Once you arrive at your home or next destination, try to open up to what happens next, with curiosity instead of having set expectations, and be kind to yourself and the people you meet.

12. Before you go to sleep, once more make time to check-in. Turn inwards to meet yourself and, if possible, allow yourself to be consciously aware of the sensation of drifting from being awake to falling asleep.

thinking individuals who, however, see in the service of their community their highest life problem."

To start on an individual level means to start with us, each of us, as an individual. If you think you are too busy, see the mindful *"can* do list" featured in the box above. It may just change your mind and give you the kick-start needed right now.

Mindfulness and corporate culture

When we see the word "corporation", our mind starts conjuring up pictures of CEOs and bankers in Docklands or on Wall Street congratulating each other for making vast amounts of money. Or of making savings by "relieving" thousands of workers of their duties. We picture meetings with boring agendas. We imagine back-room deals being made to maximize profits whilst ignoring any broader social responsibility – ignoring the rights of children (by using factories that exploit child labour), or harming the environment. Many companies still subscribe to old, unhealthy ideas about how to make money: some rely on fear to keep people on track; a few are senselessly greedy and utterly ruthless, whilst others are just clueless and self-serving, heedless of their impact on the environment and the inhabitants of the planet.

But that is far from the whole picture. For example, one global player who faced up to the times and began to act sustainably is Google. That particular extremely successful modern corporation designed a course based on emotional intelligence for its staff. One of the main aspects of that course was mindfulness – introduced by Jon Kabat-Zinn himself and then developed as an internal emotional intelligence programme by Chade-Meng Tan. The latter is Google's "unofficial greeter, its jolly good fellow" as Kabat-Zinn stated it in his foreword to Meng's book *Search Inside Yourself*. This book describes how an internal mindfulness programme can change the lives of staff and hence the company at large.

Google, a corporate giant that owns the world's most successful search engine, offers these classes to employees as a way to empower the individual. Happier employees are more engaged, make better decisions and go the extra mile that little bit more cheerfully.

It doesn't matter where or how we develop mindfulness, it doesn't matter why, and it ultimately doesn't even matter what we do. As long as it is done mindfully it is all good. Any practice or activity that supports reflection over reactivity, encourages *feeling* emotions rather than simply acting on them and opens awareness to what is really going on is of benefit. Slow down, notice and savour: that's a great way to build mental wealth. All mindfulness is good mindfulness.

This is something that you come to realize more and more as you delve deeper into your own practice. Mindfulness can come about through any activity, as long as you are aware of what you are doing when you are doing it. You could be in the most boring and mind-bendingly dull place in the world, but if you can recognise the boredom and become aware of how you feel about it you will be mindful. Remember to notice:

* What is your body doing?
* What thoughts are running through your head?

These things are always with you wherever you are. Take advantage of that simple truth. Google goes in for some surprising, quirky approaches to staff facilities. But, in addition to providing indoor massage chairs that face aquariums or huge slides between floors. Google has recognized that this sort of course will ultimately help employees in more ways than one. The fostering of a supportive environment in which mindfulness practice is encouraged could go a long way towards transforming corporate culture for the better. Whilst it is behaving in an exemplary manner towards staff in this regard, Google does still have some way to go to address broader issues of corporate responsibility in its operation in the marketplace – an example of this was its apparent collusion with the Chinese Government in limiting its search engine in China.

Hopefully, their journey towards being a mindful organisation will bring about change here too.

There are a growing number of companies building a work force that no longer has a slave mentality of submissive subordinates: individuals and groups who have their own visions, goals and insights. Humanity has changed, both individually and collectively. The last few years have witnessed uprisings against national dictators, revolts aimed at creating new structures, with democracy as their goal. Those in power are no more sovereign; they have to face the consequences if they stick to their outdated autocratic behaviour.

And what we can see happening on a political and societal level is also happening on the corporate level. The workforce has to be included instead of commanded; that is something that the leading people in many companies have still to learn. The good news is that some leaders and companies have already understood. The torch is lit.

Now even those individuals working in "mindless" companies can learn to practise mindfulness and reap the benefits of doing so. We wonder how long corporations would be able to resist if their employees built up an atmosphere of mindfulness and changed the culture of their workplaces from within. The workforce is striking back; a mindful revolution is blooming.

12

Mindfulness and personal growth

Via mindfulness, we notice the whole breadth of our life experiences. Life becomes a sensual dance of impressions – of emotions, images, urges and impulses. Through the practice, we become aware of how it affects our well-being. With practice we are able to notice the stream of life and move downstream gently with the flow, rather than feeling as though we are constantly struggling to swim upstream. We are talking here about the quality of life and how to enhance it; this is about personal growth.

Mindfulness – a journey of self-discovery

Imagine life simply unfolding, and doing so in the most surprising of ways. Rather, that is, than always pushing uphill, and getting nowhere because we do not know where we really want to go. We are unable to see our own vision for life clearly; our view of its panoramic horizons is troubled. If we are always wondering how to manage all the personal and professional dramas which assail us, in a state of anxiety, we don't recognize the clues and opportunities that present themselves to help us realize our vision. We fail to notice those revelations that pop into our mind out of nowhere: words from strangers, or from the lyrics of a song, snippets of news heard or read, or insistent fragments of experience from our own past.

The vision of life: our personal horizon

We can, right now, start to pause, to check in and listen to ourselves, to allow the curtain to be drawn aside so that we become aware of our vision for how we would like our life to be, based on our personal horizon. Wherever we are, right now in our lives, is likely to determine where our personal horizon lies. If we are worried about how to pay the rent tomorrow, how to feed the kids, how to simply survive, we are unlikely to be in a position to be concerned about global affairs – about how human beings are treated in other countries thousands of miles away, or about climate change. Our vision for our own life is limited to how to survive each day as best we can.

Or we may be comfortably off, fairly well fed, have a job and a long-term relationship. Then perhaps our horizon is different. Perhaps this allows us to see a little bit further, meaning our horizon is broader: we are able to see a vision of a future (albeit an unpredictable one).

Our perspective is related to where we are: if we are down in a deep ditch surrounded by threat, if we are on level ground, at sea level or up on a hill or mountain, our horizon will be different. Whatever our current reality is, our vision is related to our current horizon.

> *Pain is inevitable. Suffering is optional."*
> *Dalai Lama*

Physics teaches us that everything consists of frequencies – which can interfere with each other. So as we continue to focus on difficult events or impossible situations in our life, we are actually aligning the frequency at which we vibrate with some frequency of struggle and suffering, keeping us in a continuous loop. And we are attached to our suffering. It's hard to imagine, but it's true. Actually the attachment is the result of repeating the same old habits and patterns again and again. We all do it, until we decide that enough is enough and we need a different way to live. That's the moment to pause and to look up.

Pain and suffering – and not much else – occurs as a result of being constantly in our own heads. We all suffer to varying degrees from a lack of belief in ourselves. This is the unconscious mind, or the inner critic or censor undermining us, whispering things such as: "Who do you think you are? You will fail. It's not safe. Let's stay quiet and small." As children, we absorbed the disparagement of those who repeatedly told us of our inadequacies, our limitations and our unworthiness. Unfortunately our educators didn't know better. But now *we* know better.

With know-how, a commitment to practice and support, a new awareness can be created. We can open up to a simpler, more beautiful way of living, a life designed to be full of joy. So the trail changes at this crossroads. The new path is towards *self-compassion* and *self-esteem*.

Self-compassion: closely related to mindfulness

Like mindfulness, we can cultivate self-compassion through meditation practices. Self-compassion is an adaptive way of relating to the self and is associated with many aspects of psychological wellbeing. The writer and psychologist Paul Gilbert, head of the Mental Health Research Unit at the University of

Derby, has written several fascinating books on the notion and practice of self-compassion, such as *The Compassionate Mind*.

The evidence that self-compassion is a mediator of change in mindfulness-based approaches isn't as strong as for other potential mechanisms such as mindfulness itself or psychological flexibility. It is not an area which has been fully researched. However, what research does show is that mindfulness training can lead to an increase in self-compassion and that increased self-compassion is associated with improved wellbeing and healthy psychological functioning.

Self-compassion versus self-esteem

Although self-compassion may seem similar to self-esteem, they are different in many ways. Self-esteem refers to our sense of self-worth, our perceived value, or how much we like ourselves. While there is little doubt that low self-esteem is problematic and often leads to depression and lack of motivation, trying to acquire higher self-esteem can also be problematic.

In modern Western culture, self-esteem is often based on how much we differ from others, how much we stand out. It's about being special. It is not okay to be average; we have to feel above average to feel good about ourselves.

This means that attempts to raise self-esteem may also result in narcissistic, self-absorbed behaviour or lead us to put others down in order to feel better about ourselves. We may also have a tendency to get angry and aggressive towards those who have said or done anything that potentially makes us feel bad about ourselves. The need for high self-esteem may encourage us to ignore, distort or hide personal shortcomings so that we can't see ourselves clearly and accurately.

In addition, our self-esteem is often contingent on our latest success or failure, meaning that it fluctuates depending on ever-changing circumstances. In contrast to self-esteem, self-compassion is not based on self-evaluation. People feel compassion for themselves because all human beings deserve compassion and understanding, not because they possess some particular set of traits such as being clever or good-looking. This means that, with self-compassion, we don't have to feel better than others to feel good about ourselves.

Self-compassion also allows for greater self-clarity, because personal failings can be acknowledged with kindness and do not need to be hidden or denied. Moreover, self-compassion isn't dependent on external circumstances; it's always available – especially when you fail spectacularly!

Research indicates that by comparison with self-esteem, self-compassion is associated with greater emotional resilience, more accurate self-concepts, more caring behaviour in relationships, and less narcissism and reactive anger.

Exercise: self-compassion

We invite you to consider the following. Ask yourself:

* How self-compassionate are you?

* How do you typically react to yourself?

* What types of things do you typically judge and criticize yourself for (appearance, career, relationships, parenting, etc)?

* What type of language do you use with yourself when you notice some flaw or make a mistake (do you insult yourself, or do you take a more kind and understanding tone)?

* When you are being highly self-critical, how does this make you feel inside?

* When you notice something about yourself that you

don't like, do you tend to feel cut off from others, or do you feel connected with fellow humans who are also imperfect?

✱ What are the consequences of being so hard on yourself?

✱ Does it make you more motivated and happy, or discouraged and depressed?

✱ How do you think you would feel if you could truly love and accept yourself exactly as you are?

✱ Does this possibility scare you, give you hope or both?

If we have honestly reflected on these questions and have listened to ourselves carefully, we should be now forming a few ideas about our own ability to be self-compassionate.

Let the past be where it belongs – in the past!

Many experiences from the past live on in our unconscious mind. They serve to keep us mired in the past, unable to get beyond our current experience. Most of us long for peace of mind, for the confidence to live our dreams, for the capacity to make a real contribution to the world. But that nagging feeling keeps on at us – "Don't step off the beaten path: it's not safe". And any dreams we may have remain unexpressed.

We are the creator, the artist, the performer and executor of our life. We have desires for a better life with more meaning. We know that we should be acknowledging this and then letting it go. But it is the letting go and being still that most people have difficulty with. The letting go provides the freedom and space for the creative artist to bloom and the efficient performer to act.

We may not think that we are artists. But that is exactly what we are every day of our lives. We paint our future with the images, pictures and feelings that we experience today.

The problem is that we keep re-creating the same picture over and over, by seeing only what is in front of us and not exploring our vision. If life isn't looking the way we want it to be, then it's time to paint a new picture.

Can you imagine going through your day feeling wholly at ease, content with how your life is unfolding? Imagine for a minute what it would be like without all that worry and all that stress. What a relief it would be! What if we would just be still for a moment with ourselves?

Take several deep breaths and allow your body to relax. Just breathing and listening to the wisdom inside. Everything we need is right there within us. Let's stay there a little longer, relaxing.

* What do you see, hear or feel in that silence?
* What do you know or understand about the truth of who you are?
* You know you're powerful
* You know you're here to experience the joy and wonder of your life
* This is your life. Live it now. Now *is* all there is – we all only have moments to live!

When we are practising mindfulness, we are able to hear the gentle voice of our authentic self. When we are able to listen to this gentle voice, we are becoming self-compassionate.

Exercise: self-compassion 2

We invite you to consider the following. Ask yourself:

* How do you typically react to life's difficulties?
* How do you treat yourself when you run into challenges in your life?
* Do you tend to ignore the fact that you're suffering and

focus exclusively on fixing the problem? Or do you stop to give yourself some care and comfort?

* Do you tend to get carried away by the drama of the situation, so that you make a bigger deal out of it than necessary, or do you tend to keep things in perspective?

* Do you feel cut off from others when things go wrong?

* Do you ever experience the irrational feeling that everyone else is having a better time of it? Or are you in touch with the fact that all humans experience hardship in their lives?

If we feel that we lack sufficient self-compassion, we check-in with ourselves. Please don't start criticizing yourself for this too. If you are, stop right now! We are trying to feel compassion for ourselves, for how difficult life is as an imperfect human being in this extremely competitive society of ours.

We live in a culture which does not emphasize self-compassion – quite the reverse in fact. We are told that we're being lazy and self-indulgent if we are not our own harshest critic. We are told that no matter how hard we try, our best just isn't good enough. It is time for something different. We can all benefit by learning to be more self-compassionate and now is the perfect time to start.

A mindful lifestyle

Now we are not saying all problems and difficulties will cease, because they won't. What we are saying is that it will seem that you encounter nowhere near as many of them. When they do occur, you will not be destabilized by them as easily and you will be well-placed to find solutions. If you allow it, that is!

When the mind is still, we are able at last to notice all the sweet sounds, the beauty and the connections that usually pass us by so many times a day. When we move towards a mindful lifestyle, life simply flows. In our experience, life is not the struggle that it was when we were playing things over and over in our mind, trying to manage and control all this "stuff" and feeling life to be out of the control we wanted to have over it.

The truth is, *we cannot control life*. So we allow it to happen in the most wonderful way, to be surprised and uplifted and nourished by it. This can only happen when our mind is still and we surrender to and trust the power of life.

But this does not mean that we cannot plan or design our own life. When the conscious and the unconscious minds are quiet, we are free to appreciate the *vision* we have for our life. We can learn to allow our creativity to emerge day by day, recognizing our *current reality* for what it is, removing the obstacles we place in our own way and allowing life to unfold beautifully – seemingly miraculously. Then what we want to achieve, the *goals* we have to move forward with our life (those landmarks on our map towards achieving our vision) will each bring us closer to our final destination – a fulfilled life.

These concepts are at the heart of a mindfulness-based approach which we have developed: an eight-week Mindfulness-Based Awareness Coaching™ (MBAC) programme. This is intended as a continuation of the original Mindfulness-Based Stress Reduction Programme (MBSR) outlined in Chapter 10. Over the course of eight sessions, all grounded in mindfulness practice, participants are able to gain the insights they need to elaborate an individual life plan, using the V.GROWTH© coaching model. This model provides the structure for the programme, which is delivered on a foundation of both formal and informal mindfulness practices.

The V.GROWTH model

V   vision

G   goals

R   reality

O   options, opportunities and obstacles

W   the way ahead

T   task force

H   the happy hour

Our **Vision** is defined by our personal horizon – the view we have from the here and now, our awareness of what is happening around us. It's determined by where we are and by looking as far as we can see. It's the perspective we have on the future we want: our dreams of personal development. If we know our direction, if we really have defined our vision, our current **Reality** has already changed. Now we are looking forward and we are able to leave the past where it belongs – behind us!

From this perspective, we can survey the **Goals** we set ourselves to achieve our vision – the milestones in our lives – as well as the **Opportunities**, **Options** and **Obstacles** along the **Way**. And we are not alone in our travels; there are always companions with us on this journey. The moment we become aware of them, we have found our **Task Force** – those who will support us along the way. This task force remains until the job is done and we can finally evaluate the outcome honestly and celebrate our success – the **Happy Hour**. Let's look at those concepts in more detail.

Vision

Our vision is not something we will readily attain. It describes a dream, an ideal or a direction; something we are working towards. Some would call this a higher or super goal. As described previously, our vision is related to our personal horizon. This horizon expands with our own development and the same is true for our vision; it becomes more inclusive and clearer.

Unfortunately it is also true that many people have no vision for their life at all. Others do have dreams but declare them unattainable; they see them as unrealistic and hopelessly far-fetched. But that's exactly the difference between a vision and a goal.

By means of mindfulness practice we are able to discover our authentic self and through that we can discover our core values, attitudes and dreams.

If one advances confidently in the direction of his dreams, and endeavours to live the life which he has imagined, he will meet with success unexpected in common hours.
Henry David Thoreau

Goals

If the work we put in to produce a clear vision was honestly and thoroughly accomplished, our goals will be readily apparent. We can then clearly see the milestones and landmarks we have to reach and pass on our journey towards our vision. Very often the people we are coaching are extremely surprised at how easy effective goal-setting becomes when the vision is clear.

I can't change the direction of the wind, but I can adjust my sails to always reach my destination.
Jimmy Ray Dean
(Country music singer, TV host, actor and businessman)

Reality

What we mean by reality is the here and now – where we stand in life at this precise moment. This current reality is all that we really have in life: *this* moment. We all only have moments to live. How many will there be all together? Nobody knows. There are only moments – from the moment when we took our first breath to the moment we breathe our last. These moments and every moment in-between constitute our life. Through mindfulness we become aware of our options, opportunities and the obstacles which confront us – moment by moment.

> *Don't bury your thoughts – put your vision to reality.*
> *Wake up and live!*
> *Bob Marley*

Options, opportunities and obstacles

When we gather and consider our options and opportunities – when we find out what they offer, what benefits they may bring, how helpful they might be and what advantages they might have – we discover with surprise and growing self-confidence the potential we have for self-development.

No doubt we will also identify where we have deficiencies, notice our tendency to procrastinate and identify our fears and avoidance strategies – the obstacles, the barriers and the threats. But this time we will scrutinize them with curiosity instead of resentment, with a readiness to seek solutions instead of a self-fulfilling helplessness. And yes, we will also be exploring effective tools and proven techniques to transform those obstacles into manageable challenges.

> *Obstacles don't have to stop you. If you run into a wall, don't turn around and give up. Figure out how to climb it, go through it, or work around it.*
> *Michael Jordan*

The way ahead

Here we pull together everything we've learned to date and create an "action plan" to realize our desired outcomes – be that a plan for a fulfilling life, a successful enterprise, or a sustainable project. And we do it mindfully, from the inception of the plan until its realization.

In making any plan, we seek to remain conscious of the consequences for ourselves, the people around us, the environment we are in and so on. Being aware of the consequences of what we do is, of course, applied mindfulness.

We do make a difference - one way or the other. We are responsible for the impact of our lives. Whatever we do with whatever we have, we leave behind us a legacy for those who follow.
Stephen Covey (author of The Seven Habits of Highly Effective People)

Task force

We do not have to set out alone on the journey to realize our action plan. There are always companions on the road; they may be temporary, and only along for one leg of the journey, or they may be there for the whole trip. If we use our newly gained self-confidence we only have to look around us to become aware of people who will offer support, key influencers, mentors or coaches.

In particular, we may be able to identify someone who will offer closer support – who will perhaps oversee and monitor our progress. If we make our plan public to somebody we trust and that person is willing to become our sounding board and constructive critic, they can ask the clarifying questions and challenge our progress in a positive way.

With this support we will stay on track or become aware when a change of direction is needed. All plans are likely to require some amendments, some reorientations at various points during their realization. That is in the nature of action plans and these adjustments ensure their successful completion.

> *Tell everyone what you want to do and*
> *someone will want to help you do it.*
> **William Clement Stone** *(American businessman,*
> *philanthropist and author)*

Happy hour

Finally, we evaluate the outcome of our adventure. We explore what went well, which elements were successful and what goals we have achieved. We look at the reasons we succeeded and how we did so. These positive results should *always* be celebrated.

And what about the mistakes and failures? We analyse these as well and we do so thoroughly because they offer us a chance to learn. Without mistakes and failures we don't have the opportunity to discover what we can do differently when we have a comparable situation. This in itself is a reason to celebrate.

These are the moments which refuel our motivational tanks with the energy needed when we set out again to face future challenges. As we have outlined in previous chapters, every personal development influences our direct and broader environment. It always starts with personal growth.

> *We are all inventors, each sailing out on a voyage of discovery, guided each by a private chart, of which there is no duplicate. The world is all gates, all opportunities.*
> *Ralph Waldo Emerson*

PART FOUR

Mindfulness at large

13

Mindfulness, religion, the spirit

Mindfulness practices have been applied to human endeavours for thousands of years. They have been found to be of great value by Hindus, Buddhists, Muslims, Christians and others; across Asia, Europe and the Americas; and in the distant past, in the Middle Ages and in modern times.

The depth and breadth of human experience with mindfulness practices in itself argues very powerfully for their intrinsic worth in solving problems in our inner experience, which is arguably the métier of clinical psychology.

The following overview explores the similarities and differences between these major traditions, all of which are linked to mindfulness in one way or another.

Hinduism and mindfulness

The beginnings of Hinduism have been dated to as far back as 1000 BC. Hinduism has no single historical founder, but its tradition teaches that its spiritual laws and truths were revealed to spiritual men ("rishis") and women ("rishikas"), who lived along the banks of the Ganges and Indus rivers in northern India.

Central to Hinduism is the concept of Brahman: a universal spirit that is the origin and support of the universe. Brahman is the supreme, absolute, eternal, infinite, spirit being. The word has been variously translated as "God", "Godhead", or "the ground of existence". Hinduism teaches that only that which is permanent is real and, because all things are subject to change except Brahman, only Brahman is real. There is a large pantheon of Hindu deities, but all are seen as different aspects of the one Brahman.

According to Hinduism, every living thing has a spirit or soul, called an "atman", which comes from Brahman. The final destination of the human soul is union with Brahman, but this cannot be achieved in just one lifetime. Therefore each individual atman, or soul, must pass from body to body, lifetime after lifetime, guided by the law of "karma". The term karma means deed or act and the law broadly refers to the universal principle of cause and effect. Rather than referring to fate or predetermination, according to the law of karma our actions can mitigate the effects experienced. Reincarnation or the transmigration of the soul is subject to this law, which determines what type of life will be lived in each reincarnation; our current life is the product of our deeds in past lives, and our next reincarnation will depend on our deeds in this one.

Hinduism is the birthplace of virtually all Asian contemplative traditions. The Sanskrit word "yoga" (which can be translated as "discipline") applies to a wide range of contemplative practices designed to eventually unite the individual atman with Brahman. Hinduism evolved to preach not asceticism or renunciation, but rather a more complicated form of enlightenment – namely yoga. Whereas Buddhism has spawned movements such as Zen, encouraging the cessation of action to find mindfulness, Hinduism asks its followers to be yogis or skilful in action. What Hinduism says is that by practising meditation and being mindful during everyday actions, eventually we can find time for meditation no matter what we do (informal practice): we can meditatively work at the office, we can meditatively play basketball, we can meditatively survive morning rush hour. We'll come to live in the present, free from the distractions of the mind, without the fear of having to give up the world and its attachments.

Buddhism and mindfulness

The religion of Buddhism was founded in India by Siddhartha Gautama, later called "the Buddha", who lived between 560 and 480 BC. Siddhartha Gautama was raised in an affluent family and did not even know that poverty existed until he left the pleasant confines of his father's palace. Siddhartha was so disturbed by the poverty and despair that he witnessed that he decided to go on a spiritual journey to find answers to the questions this suffering had provoked in him. Shaving his head and donning a robe, Siddhartha Gautama travelled and consulted with gurus and spiritual teachers.

Finally, Siddhartha began to meditate, became enlightened and developed a teaching that became known as the Noble Eightfold path. The path leads to nirvana or "perfect insight" – not a heaven, but a quality of mind. The method is mindfulness, the expression is compassion and the essence is wisdom. These eight techniques consisted of:

* right belief
* right aspiration

* right speech
* right action
* right occupation
* right effort
* right thought
* right meditation

Buddhist mindfulness techniques centre on seated meditation and mindfulness of the breath. One of the oldest Buddhist meditation practices is "vipassana" (discernment) meditation, which is a graded, deeply intellectual system of attempting to directly perceive the truths of the body, feelings, consciousness and the objects of the mind. The most familiar Buddhist meditation system is probably Zen, the Japanese version of Mahayana Buddhist teaching. It places less importance on knowledge of doctrine in favour of direct understanding through "zazen" ("seated meditation"). It is undertaken in order to calm the body and the mind: via intense concentration, a meditator gains insight into the nature of existence, and eventually reaches enlightenment.

Taoism/Daoism and mindfulness

Laozi (or Lao Tzu) is traditionally regarded as the founder of Taoism (later on called Daoism). He is closely associated in this context with original (sometimes known as "primordial") Taoism and is revered as a deity. Whether he actually existed is widely disputed; there are references to him being a contemporary of Confucius, an official and a historian. The work attributed to him – the *Daodejing* – dates to the late fourth century BC.

Taoism draws its cosmological foundations from the concept of "Yinyang" (as do many different schools of Chinese thought). In Chinese philosophy, Yin is the principle of darkness, negativity and femininity, the counterpart of Yang which is the principle of light, motivation and masculinity. These two opposite yet complementary principles are thought to exist in varying proportions in all things.

From its beginnings, Taoism has concerned itself with creating a harmonious relationship between humans and the natural the world through direct contemplation of the "ground of existence" – that which remains after all objects are extinguished. The ground of existence, the system of the world and the method of achieving harmony are all terms by which the Chinese term "dao" can be translated. Taoism's best-known contributions to mindfulness practice are Qigong exercises – in which breath and movement are aligned and placed at the heart of exercise, healing and meditation – and the martial art Tai Chi Chuan, or the "Daoist Fist". Both are movement-based meditation systems.

Christianity and mindfulness

The Christian contemplative tradition flowered in the Middle Ages with the introduction, in about 530 CE, of coenobitic (communal) monasteries. Among the great Christian mystics of this period are St John of the Cross, who coined the famous and poetic term "dark night of the soul"; St Teresa de Ávila, who described a seven-stage visionary journey to the throne of God; and St Hildegard of Bingen, who wrote chants and songs based upon her inner experiences. For several centuries after the rise of Protestantism, the mystical tradition and its insistence on a direct, imminent experience of God fell out of favour.

It was, however, kept alive by smaller nonconformist traditions such as Quakerism until the rise of Pentecostal

Christianity in the nineteenth century. Several mainstream Christian churches have rediscovered the medieval mystics in an attempt to compete with Pentecostalism in feeding their parishioners' need for a more direct, personal experience of God. Mindfulness, in a Christian context, is an awakened state of thought and mind, which recognizes that in God and Jesus "we live and move and have our being" (Acts 17:28). It is the practice of discovering the presence of God: living mindfully, for a Christian, is living from and in the God-Presence within.

Judaism and mindfulness

As with Christianity, the Middle Ages also saw the birth of Jewish contemplative practices, the most famous of which is Kabbala, meaning "received tradition". It's a practice that centres on a very close reading of Jewish scripture with reference to a system of numerological relations.

The student of Kabbala enters into a deep contemplation of the relationships between verses, words, letters and their numerological equivalents, creating a powerful web of associational meaning across them all, which points to a mystical, immanent understanding of the divine. Like the Christian mystical tradition, Kabbala has enjoyed a renewed popularity in the US in recent years.

Sufism and mindfulness

Like Christianity and Judaism, Islam developed a mystical tradition well after its foundation (in about 610 CE). It was not until the ninth century CE that the tradition of Sufism emerged out of a reaction to a growing legalism in Islam. The heart of Sufism is a search for a direct confrontation with the divine, often described as love or symbolized as an all-consuming fire.

Sufism employs a fantastic variety of techniques, but the most familiar of these is that practised by the Persian Mevlevi-ye order – the moving meditation of the whirling dervishes in which the practitioner whirls for hours steadily anti-clockwise on the left foot, with the right arm high, palm skyward, and the left arm down, palm earthward.

This distinctive practice is a visualization of the movement of the world, with God in the still centre and energy coming down from heaven and into the earth through the body of the whirler.

The Osho movement and mindfulness

Osho (1931–90) was born in Madhya Pradesh, India. A meditation practitioner and teacher, his birth name was Chandra Mohan Jain but he was probably best known under the name Bhagwan Shree Rajneesh during the 1970s. He became a professor of philosophy at Jabalpur University, and resigned in 1966 to become a spiritual teacher in his own right, initiating his disciples as "Sannyasins". In the 1970s he started attracting Westerners and in 1981 he moved his community to Oregon in the US (where it became infamous partly on account of Osho's fleet of 93 Rolls Royces). His life-affirmative teachings attracted a certain amount of international fame for their enjoyment and celebration of the body and sexuality. In 1985 the commune was disbanded after Osho was arrested and charged with a number of crimes including immigration offences. He was acquitted but deported, returning to Pune where the movement flourished until his death, and where it still continues.

Despite his colourful personal history, his teachings are valuable. In their essence, they are against all doctrine and

Vipassana meditation

Vipassana meditation is often also described as "mindfulness meditation" or "insight meditation". Unfortunately the word mindfulness can be a bit misleading if we are interpreting mindfulness simply to mean that we are constantly thinking about what we're doing. "Mindful" in the proper sense of the word means to be attentive to and conscious about what's happening.

The word insight can be a little misleading too because it's not only a word used in Buddhism, but also in psychotherapy. When we successfully engage in psychotherapy we receive insights. Of course those insights are very important, but they are typically insights into our own personality, and the specific issues of our life. The insights that come as a result of vipassana are both deeper and more general than those that are ordinarily encountered in psychotherapy. In science, a deep theory allows many specific applications. In the same way, the insights that come from mindfulness practice let us understand the very nature of personality itself, not just things about our own personality. So vipassana refers to "insight" in the sense of deep insight and it is "mindfulness" in the sense of extraordinary attentiveness.

belief and teach that the aim of spiritual development is enlightenment. One prerequisite for this is to become free of all socialization, through a comprehensive programme of traditional and newly invented meditations, and a range of therapies. His ideas are eclectic, drawing on the mystical traditions of all of the world's religions as well as many modern mystics, and seek to integrate Eastern and Western techniques.

He said that whatever we do, we should do it mindfully: we should be mindful when we talk, when we walk and even when we blink. We should do nothing senselessly, unconsciously; whatever we do simply because it is fashionable will lead invariably to transgression. Whatever we do without awareness leads us away from ourselves; the only method of coming close to our self is to become more and more aware.

Whatever the circumstances and whatever the situation, we should hold fast and never let go of our awareness. Even if we stand to lose everything; even if our house catches fire, we should move only with complete awareness.

Transcendental meditation

In this guide to mindfulness we should also have a look at the main "competitor" in the battle to win over both meditation novice and the scientists' favour.

Many people in the West receive their first exposure to meditation through what we know as transcendental meditation or TM. TM is essentially the classic mantra practice of India, but presented by the Maharishi Mahesh Yogi in a contemporary format, one that is accessible to Westerners.

Maharishi Mahesh Yogi, often known simply as "Maharishi" or "The Maharishi" was born around 1918 – his exact date of birth is uncertain – and passed away in 2008. In the summer of 1967, the year of Flower Power, he made headlines when the four Beatles, with their wives and girlfriends, as well as Mick Jagger, Jane Asher and Marianne Faithfull, followed the Maharishi from London to Bangor in Wales to sit very publicly at his feet supporting his message of universal love and peace.

Although the Maharishi's more grandiose claims to be saving the world through transcendental meditation and other spiritual techniques such as levitation or "flying" attracted ridicule as well as curiosity, he was shrewdly aware that publicity, however negative, could be used to gain converts and to broaden his base of recruitment.

Known from his early days in India as the "giggling guru" because of his sparkling eyes and bubbling witticisms, Mahesh succeeded in making TM his personal trademark, netting for his organization assets that came to be measured in billions.

While he never abandoned his claim to be transforming humanity's consciousness in the direction of universal harmony and peace, he built a highly successful empire out of selling the spiritual techniques practised by his followers and used by companies as aids to stress management.

Executives who learned to meditate often found their performance and productivity improved, and so large corporations such as IBM and Toyota had no more objections to sending staff on transcendental meditation courses than they had about the development of other personal skills.

Mindfulness versus TM

On the surface mindfulness and TM would seem to be very different, perhaps even antithetical. Typically in TM, a meditator leans back against a wall, withdraws from the phenomenal world and repeats a mantra for perhaps twenty minutes. It is relatively easy for a novice to engage in this practice and often brings immediate calming effects.

In mindfulness practice – as we have learned – we sit upright, standing or lying down, with intense alertness, attending to the flow of ordinary experience. This usually means focusing on rather banal and sometimes uncomfortable phenomena such as itches, sounds, thought patterns, pains and the like. It would almost seem that the mantra practice "takes us out" while the mindfulness practice "brings us in".

However, beneath the surface differences, these two practices have much in common that can easily go unrecognized.

For one thing, both practices build calm and concentration, albeit in different ways. In mantra practice, the meditator relaxes, withdraws and lets the rhythmic sounds of a mantra replace the chaotic sounds of internal conversations. This develops concentration, since "internal chatter" is the major source of distraction in daily life.

In mindfulness practice, we hold each moment of ordinary experience in awareness. Awareness soaks into our thoughts like water into a sponge. In effect this represents a kind of silent merging with each phenomenon as it arises in the six senses – hearing, seeing, smelling, tasting, the feeling body and the thinking mind.

Mantras, as used in TM, are repetitive rhythms. They set up periodic waves or vibrations in our consciousness. Imagine a pool of water in which very regular, pleasing patterns of ripples continuously spread outwards from the centre across the water. Focusing on those ripples could easily take you into a state of relaxation. This is one facet of how mantra works. Its repetitive nature sets up rhythmic ripples throughout the meditator's whole consciousness. The meditator then focuses on the regularity of those ripples and rides them into deeper and deeper levels of relaxation, concentration and integration.

In mindfulness practice we focus on a sequence of sensory objects, but because of the penetrating way we are focusing on them these objects sometimes vanish almost as soon as they arise. Buddhists call this impermanence.

Should we then consider mindfulness to be a better form of meditation than employing mantras? Not at all! Such simple comparisons between meditation techniques are not appropriate. Each way of meditating has its own characteristic strong points and weak points. And we all have our personal needs and preferences.

Mantra practice is easy to start with and has – at least theoretically – the potential to influence daily life. Mindfulness practice can be difficult if not downright painful, especially at the beginning. By way of compensation it equips us with a systematic procedure that will transform any ordinary experience of daily life into a profound contact with our authentic self.

Mindfulness and spiritual health

Love, kindness, compassion, good health and liberation from suffering are core human desires which religions and spiritual traditions all over the world have focused on since the beginning of civilization.

We have always known that those qualities are good for us, that they are essential remedies for humanity in pain. What is different now is that we have a new and powerful ally in humanity's road towards wisdom. We live in an extraordinary time, where the neurosciences, genetics, modern psychology, anthropology, physics and mathematics have converged to shed new light on what were previously seen as purely spiritual insights. The findings of neuroscience routinely endorse the claim that compassion and kindness are at the heart of health and wellbeing, which in turn are at the heart of spiritual fulfilment.

To meet the challenge of finding effective ways of embodying the principles that afford us health and wellbeing, modern neuroscience and spiritual traditions have converged to offer systematic ways of analysing what gets in the way of such liberation.

Whilst differences in cultural, historical and geographical contexts will give rise to differences in the words and metaphors used to engage in that analysis, its core structure is always and everywhere fundamentally the same, consisting of diagnosis, aetiology, prognosis and prescription.

Diagnosis – or what is wrong with us

Modern neuroscience has opened up the possibility that we can harness the power of the mind to rewire the brain by approaching the human organism very differently from the way we have done in the past. Instead of perceiving the organism as a fixed entity, we can look more deeply at its *energetic* nature – the fact that we are made of energy flows, frequencies or waves. Instead of merely diagnosing an individual as ill (or worse, "defective"), we can notice how these waves behave. Suffering may come down to energy flows not being integrated: there is an imbalance, a misalignment in the flow of energy. This certainly explains why we might feel like we are off-centre, always in the wrong place.

Neuroscience may use the language of energy flow and integration (or a lack of it). Psychology speaks of tension or relaxation on the somatic level, attunement (or lack thereof) on the emotional level and personal significance on the cognitive level (the sense we make of our life history). In the language of contemporary mind/body/spirit texts, we might speak of being in harmony (or, in contrast, out of sync) with "the source", "ultimate reality" or "spirit". And in religion, similar conditions are expressed as feeling close to, or far away from, God.

Whichever discipline or belief system's terminology is used, there is evidently a widespread diagnosis of suffering as a "being out of balance". Recognizing this is the first step towards an improvement in our individual lives and the human condition at large. This entails a curious, open and accepting acknowledgement of all the elements of suffering by not masking it, pushing it away or hiding from it. We need to accept our suffering kindly and without aggression, so that we can open ourselves to being with it, honouring it and healing it.

Aetiology – or understanding the cause of illness

How can you treat a disease if you don't know its origins and mechanisms? There are always reasons and causes for our suffering: it has origins we need to recognize and understand, but our minds play amazing tricks on us.

To put it simply, the cause of our suffering is the fact that we oversimplify reality in general and the way our organism works in particular. When we oversimplify, we distort reality and fall into ignorance.

The human organism is very complex, and we have the unique ability to be aware of being aware, to think about thinking. This means that we have the brain power to create and destroy, to be honest or to lie, to see clearly or distort, and to be in tune with nature and our bodies or go against them.

Any organism's fundamental physical drive is to ensure homeostasis (a state of equilibrium) and survival. We don't have to do anything to support that – it just happens on its own, automatically. Most of us don't have the faintest clue how pervasively this automatism controls all of our functions, from maintenance of essential bodily functions through to thinking and action. So here we have the paradox that whilst we have the power to create and destroy, as outlined above, we are also usually in autopilot mode; this creates a clouded view of reality, with distortions of truth, illusions and a false sense of what freedom really is.

There's a much-used metaphor for this state of being, borrowed from the horror movie: that we are the living dead, zombies who are unaware of being on autopilot. What's more, our ignorance about our brain's and mind's clever distortions is really no different from suffering itself – suffering is this kind of ignorance.

If we are able to see our suffering clearly, to recognize its causal mechanisms, we can start to understand possible ways out of this dilemma: a process that strengthens our intention to let go of the causes of suffering.

This letting go is the beginning of an awakening...

Being awake and being aware is the core concern of health, spirituality and religion, because we are only able to love, have compassion, heal and liberate our world from suffering when we do not allow our mind's secretions to cloud and distort our view. With awareness, our actions start to become liberating and creative.

This awareness, as we have to discover, reveals the most unexpected reality, which is that the mind's tricks prevent us from living fully, unaware of the pregnant promise of our existence.

Prognosis: future health

Freedom from suffering is possible. This insight challenges us to embark on the path of liberation, to take the medicine needed to treat the disease of imbalance and suffering. When we start working with this prognosis, with the good news, so to speak, we come to realize something even more fundamental than the causes of our suffering.

We discover that the containment of suffering, that health, wellbeing and ease, are already available to us, if we know how to recognize when they are present and enjoy the precious gifts we already have.

As we develop a deep understanding of this fact, we recognize that suffering is not as fundamental as we thought. We need to remember that, as the Dalai Lama says: "Pain is inevitable, suffering is optional". By looking deeply at our present situation, we can see that the conditions for health, integration and happiness are already there; and then we can begin to nourish these conditions.

So we come full circle. In facing our suffering and accepting it in a loving way – resisting it would only intensify it – we come to the realization that this acceptance itself is an aspect of health, ease and wellbeing and that all the conditions for ease are already there to be lived. In other words, suffering and happiness are not separate, but one and the same.

The prescription

We really do now have to start practising in a pragmatic and creative manner. Our practice is not like a musician practising on an instrument, although there are similarities to this. It is about being in the moment, on purpose, as if our lives depended on it. It is more like a vocation, like a doctor practising medicine. The word vocation derives from the Latin "vox", meaning voice. The use of the term here is deliberate; to commit to this practice of being alive is to send forth our voice into the world, to declare in no uncertain terms how deeply committed we are to alleviating suffering in ourselves and all around us.

So this prescription – to practice – also entails a number of precise instructions that are all encompassed by the discipline of mindfulness meditation. This "spiritual" discipline is deeply grounded in modern science, which informs our understanding about the way the brain and the body work. We are enormously complex organisms, and require equally complex, refined and skilful means to address the problems created by who we are.

Nature, spirituality and interconnectedness

It is in the ordinariness – of life and of the organism that we are – that we discover how extraordinary nature is. Embedded in the anatomy of the human brain is a unique structure not found in any other living creature on this planet, the medial prefrontal cortex (MPC). This MPC not only gives us the gift of consciousness, but also a whole collection of capabilities: morality, insight, empathy, intuition, compassion and, yes, mindfulness. These can transform us from a destructive species to one able to live in harmony with our earth.

Over the course of evolution we became knowing organisms, acquiring a self-consciousness which allowed us to discover and understand the world we live in. But our task is to learn that all of this knowledge is only valuable to the extent to which it is put to the service of compassion. It follows that the highest form of knowledge is love; understanding the true meaning of this entails a very long journey indeed.

The problem is that we are powerful, conscious beings who live by and large on autopilot, destroying the habitat we live in, rather than fully exploiting all we are capable of. The latter requires attention and effort.

Consciousness in itself is not enough. Awareness does not present us with a direction; indeed, it may lead to self-destruction. What we need is mindful awareness and that requires training. Jon Kabat-Zinn, in addressing the meaning of the word "spiritual" suggested that perhaps it means "simply experiencing wholeness and interconnectedness directly, seeing that individuality and totality are interwoven, that nothing is separate or extraneous and that everything is spiritual in the deepest sense, as long as we are there for it." We must relate to *all existence* with the humility that comes from realizing that all we need is the love and compassion necessary to overcome suffering.

The long journey of mindfulness: from the East to the West

Mindfulness is not concerned with anything transcendent or divine. It serves as an antidote to theism, a cure for sentimental piety, a scalpel for excising the tumour of metaphysical belief.
Stephen Batchelor

Mindfulness is an approach that is the result of a process of modernization, Westernization, re-interpretation, re-imagining, revitalization and reform that has been taking place not only in the West but also in Asian countries for over a century. It has been fashioned by modernizing Asian Buddhists who are deeply engaged in creating mindful responses to the dominant problems and questions of modernity such as: war, environmental destruction, conflicts between science and religion, religious pluralism, nihilism and a lack of certainty about the nature of knowledge.

What scholars have often meant by secularized mindfulness is a facet of a more global network of movements that are not the exclusive product of one geographic or cultural setting. In fact, the interest in mindfulness began in a context not of mutual curiosity, cultural exchange and open-minded ecumenical dialogue, but of competition, crisis and the violence of colonialism.

A crucial part of modernization, whether we are talking about trade or religion, is its tendency toward globalization, a tendency that in many cases compromises local diversity. In addition, modernization tends to elevate reason, experience and intuition over tradition. It champions the reinterpretation, adaptation or even outright rejection of traditional beliefs and practices on the basis of individual judgement. Religion becomes more individualized – a matter of personal choice. We adopt the right to choose and even construct our own personal religion.

Psychoanalysis and demythologization

The process of trying to distil or reconstruct meanings from teachings embedded in ancient world views is sometimes referred to as demythologization. In this regard psychoanalysis has certainly aided in the de-mythologization of Buddhism and its key approach, mindfulness. An early Western Buddhist sympathizer, Carl Theodor Strauss (1852–1937), claimed that "genuine Buddhism is the reverse of the mystical: it rejects miracles, is founded on reality and refuses to speculate about the absolute and other so-called first causes."

The translation of Buddhism into psychoanalytic language was also a significant element in the introduction of Zen Buddhism to the West, beginning with Daisetz Teitaro Suzuki's *Introduction to Zen Buddhism* (1934) for which Carl Jung, who was very interested in Eastern philosophy, wrote an appreciative preface. Later, the psychoanalyst Erich Fromm, collaborating with Suzuki, suggested that Zen was a kind of radical psychoanalysis that sought to unearth the whole of the unconscious and bring it to consciousness, thereby overcoming alienation and bringing the practitioner to wholeness.

The rise of meditation

If psychoanalysis has aided in the demythologization of Buddhism and its key approach – mindfulness – recent practical psychotherapies have helped to de-traditionalize it as well. This has led to a blossoming of the use of meditation in non-Buddhist therapeutic settings, often for non-Buddhist goals and without requiring commitment to explicitly Buddhist values. Rather than being an integral part of monastic life, bound up with its rituals, ethics and cosmology, meditation has become something not only for lay Buddhists but for those of any religion – or those who follow none at all.

Buddhism and science

The first Asians to present Buddhism to the West boldly proclaimed its essential compatibility with science. Soen Shaku (1859–1919) was one of Buddhism's best ambassadors. He was a representative of the Japanese delegation to the 1893 World's Parliament of Religions in Chicago and became the first monk to teach Zen in the US outside of immigrant communities. He was one of the most important early founders of Buddhism in the modern West.

But perhaps the most important early Western figure who attempted to interpret Buddhism through science was Paul Carus (1852–1919), who had a lifelong working partnership with Shaku. Carus was a pioneer of interfaith dialogue but is of particular importance here because of his popular presentation of a definitively rationalist, scientific Buddhist philosophy. Whilst he remained a strong sympathizer with Buddhist ideas, Carus did not commit to Buddhism or any other faith. Instead he promoted his view that a new religion, not yet fully formed, was emerging through the rise of science and increasing contact among the world's religions.

Rather than thinking of science as being a human invention, Carus perceived it as merely revealed by humanity: "science is stem and unalterable; it is a revelation which cannot be invented but must be discovered". He often insisted that scientific truth and religious truth are one and the same; truth being the correspondence of ideas and reality, irrespective of whether the path to it was scientific or religious.

For Carus, if a religion was to have any claim to truth, that truth must also be scientific. Recognizing the disjunction between these two apparently disparate ways to interpret the world, Carus and subsequent religious modernizers recast significant religious concepts as having allegorical or symbolic meaning.

Meditation often serves as a focal point for this stance, as some writers posit it as being both a scientific endeavour and a corrective to what they consider to be the excessive rationalism, materialism and reductionism of mainstream science.

At the moment, mindfulness is receiving a great deal of prestigious and positive scientific attention. But what if further scientific studies show that meditation is actually not nearly as effective in diminishing destructive emotions as, say, cognitive behavioural therapy or psychotropic medicines? Well, we need to be aware that mindfulness meditation does not necessarily need be construed as a science in order to be beneficial. Indeed, confining meditation within the discourse of scientific rationalism may leave some of its possibilities concealed.

Making the world remarkable

More than anything, mindfulness has much in common with modernist sensibilities in literature, film and art in general. Modernist literature has placed new value upon the details of everyday life in its finely tuned descriptions of the flow of consciousness and its reverence for ordinary objects and their capacity to reflect the universal. Mindfulness provides a distinctively modernist way of returning a sense of the sacred to the world without resort to the supernatural.

But what is it about this modern period that has provided an arena for mindfulness to emerge on a much broader stage, appealing to such a wide swathe of the population? One of the key features of modernity, and one so deeply ingrained that it is hard to see it, is a new kind of world-affirming attitude that began with the Reformation.

The power to re-create the familiar so that the everyday world becomes remarkable, and the recovery of the immediacy, freshness and vividness of things which had been obscured by habit and fixed conceptions, have been crucial to the literary and artistic sensibilities of the twentieth century.

At the same time, one of the consequences of postmodern globalization has been that mindfulness has been taken from its traditional sites and re-embedded in a wide variety of discourses, including those of the environmental movement and within recent dialogues between world religions. It has also become a part of the market, a "commodity" that is the basis of mindfulness courses, retreats and seminars compete with mindfulness books, CDs, apps and other online offers.

This reformulation of mindfulness in the languages of Western modernity could have two potentially opposite effects. It could accommodate itself so completely to mainstream Western values and assumptions that it no longer is an alternative to them. And so it would entirely surrender the resources it has for critiquing them.

However, it could position mindfulness in such a way that it could bring novel conceptual resources to the West. It could offer the modern world new perspectives on some of our personal, social, political and environmental problems. Indeed, if it does not speak the language of modernity, how can it even begin to address these ills?

14

The mindfulness community

Mindfulness has become a global movement; all over the world there are people practising together and sharing their experiences, either face to face or on social media platforms and forums. If we search the Internet with terms such as "mindfulness community", "mindfulness society" or "mindfulness groups" we are inundated with seemingly endless results. We can find out about a huge variety of mindful encounter options, from Buddhist "sanghas" (meditation groups) to non-religious mindfulness classes.

These figures are illustrative of the phenomenal growth of the mindfulness community – we are definitely not alone! This community is also very active in sharing and exchanging information: there are internet platforms with chat rooms and blogs, testimonials about events, teachers and a whole world of (admittedly not always) mindful communication.

So let's go on an excursion to some of the remarkable places which offer support, guidance and even leadership to members of the mindfulness community.

There are a number of general websites that are excellent resources for finding more information about mindfulness.

Be mindful www.bemindful.co.uk

This is a mindfulness website maintained by the UK's Mental Health Foundation. It contains information about MBSR and MBCT programmes, provides an online course and has a quick "stress test" that you can try.

Mindful www.mindful.org

Mindful is a US media initiative from the Foundation for a Mindful Society. In collaboration with the Hemera Foundation, Mindful supports the practice and development of mindfulness, awareness, and compassion in all aspects of modern life.

University-based mindfulness centres

Many universities throughout the world have established centres for mindfulness. Here are some of the key players on the academic stage.

CFM www.umassmed.edu/cfm/home/index

The birthplace of the mindfulness movement as we know it today is sited in the US near Boston, at the Worcester Campus of the University of Massachusetts (UMASS). This is home to the Center for Mindfulness in Medicine, Health Care, and Society (CFM), where it all began.

The CFM is the visionary force and global leader in mind–body medicine. For more than thirty years, the CFM has pioneered the integration of mindfulness meditation and other mindfulness-based approaches (MBAs) in mainstream medicine and healthcare via research, patient care and academic, medical and professional education. It has also made inroads into broader society through diverse outreach and public service initiatives.

Founded in 1995 by Jon Kabat-Zinn, PhD, the centre has been directed by Saki F. Santorelli since 2000 and is an outgrowth of the acclaimed Stress Reduction Clinic.

UCSD health.ucsd.edu/specialties/mindfulness

There is also a remarkable group of researchers located in sunny California, who are scrutinizing the evolution of MBAs following on from, or modifying, MBSR for special target groups or applications. The UCSD Center for Mindfulness, at the University of California, San Diego, offers a multi-faceted programme of clinical care, professional training, education, research and outreach intended to further the practice and integration of mindfulness into the lives of individuals throughout the healthcare and educational system, including patients, healthcare providers, students, teachers and business people.

There is a range of interesting research papers available on the UCSD website. We recommend that you browse the UCSD virtual home site and watch a video called "Mindfulness and Medicine" by the UCSD Center for Mindfulness' Director, Dr. Steven Hickman.

OMC www.oxfordmindfulness.org

The Oxford Mindfulness Centre (OMC) is an international centre of excellence within the Oxford University's Department of Psychiatry (UK) that works with partners around the world to prevent depression and enhance human potential through the therapeutic use of mindfulness. Here, Mark Williams, Zindel Segal and John Peacock combined cognitive behaviour therapy (CBT) with Jon Kabat-Zinn's MBSR and so shaped MBCT.

The OMC carries out research into the efficacy of mindfulness and its underlying mechanisms; it has programmes of education and training in mindfulness-based interventions and provides mindfulness courses within the National Health Service and for the general public.

CMRP www.bangor.ac.uk/mindfulness/centreinfo

The Centre for Mindfulness Research and Practice (CMRP) is committed to the promotion of wellbeing through the application of MBAs. The CMRP works to achieve this by training professionals in the application of MBAs and researching applications of mindfulness. It also teaches classes in MBSR and MBCT to specific populations and the general public both locally and further afield.

The CMRP (of the School of Psychology at Bangor University) offers two part-time degree courses. Rebecca Crane, current director of the CMRP, heads research into a variety of areas such as MBCT for people with cancer and their carers, mindfulness-based teacher training, mindfulness in education, mindfulness in the workplace, the implementation of MBCT into the National Health Service, and mindfulness in a parenting context.

Besides these, there are a growing number of universities and academic research institutes with very interesting websites, as well as a growing number of both commercial and not-for-profit providers servicing the demands of "mindfulness consumers".

The mindfulness market place

The Internet showcases a very diverse range – in both product range and quality – of mindfulness events and services. On offer are eight-week programmes in groups, retreats ranging from one day to a week or longer, individual coaching, therapeutic treatments and tailor-made corporate projects.

To be on the safe side, it is best to check if providers are genuinely and demonstrably committed to professional good practice standards and guidelines. These guidelines can be accessed by visiting:

UK Network for Mindfulness-Based Teacher Trainers
mindfulnessteachersuk.org.uk

CFM: training teachers to deliver MBSR
www.umassmed.edu/cfm/trainingteachers/index.aspx

The principles and standards for the training of teachers to deliver mindfulness-based approaches (MBAs) have been developed over the past ten years by a cohort of senior teachers and teacher-trainers in America and Europe.

This self-regulatory framework, consisting of guidelines, standards and good practice commitments, is meant to be a collection of living documents – revised, refined and articulated more fully over time through the contribution of teachers and teacher-trainers worldwide.

Books

From our personal and professional point of view, there are some must-read books out there. Some are established classics and some were published more recently. Here are a select few titles for further reading.

Full Catastrophe Living Jon Kabat-Zinn *Piatkus Press*

The first title goes without saying. No mindfulness reading list would be complete without Jon Kabat-Zinn's book on MBSR. Since its initial publication in 1990, *Full Catastrophe Living* has sold over 400,000 copies worldwide. It has established itself both as an excellent beginner's guide to meditation and as the bible of a mind/body movement that has transformed Western medicine.

This practical, step-by-step meditation guide is based on MBSR and the latest edition includes a new introduction from Jon, with a review of how MBSR has developed over the years, along with an expanded bibliography and resources section.

Wherever You Go, There You Are Jon Kabat-Zinn *Piatkus Press*

Another masterpiece from Jon. "Mindfulness," he writes, "is considered the heart of Buddhist meditation, but its essence is universal and of deep practical benefit to everyone." In this book he maps out a simple path for cultivating mindfulness in our lives and awakening us to the unique beauty and possibilities of each present moment. He shows us how this simple meditation technique can enable us to be truly in touch with where we already are, so that we can be fully aware at all times. Jon explains what mindfulness is; how to achieve mindfulness using simple meditation techniques; how mindful meditation can enhance every aspect of your life; and how to incorporate mindfulness into your everyday routine. Our recommendation is that you read *Full Catastrophe Living* first and continue the journey with *Wherever You Go, There You Are.*

The Mindful Way Through Depression Mark Williams, John Teasdale, Zindel Segal and Jon Kabat-Zinn *Guilford Press*

This book draws on the collective wisdom of four internationally renowned mindfulness experts to provide effective relief from the most prevalent psychological disorder – depression. It describes an authoritative, easy-to-use self-help programme, based on methods clinically proven to reduce the recurrence of depression and to reveal the hidden psychological mechanisms that cause chronic unhappiness. The authors gently guide readers through a series of exercises designed to break the mental habits that lead to despair.

Mindfulness: A Practical Guide to finding Peace in a Frantic World Mark Williams and Danny Penman *Piatkus Press*

The book talks about the kind of happiness that gets into our bones. It seeps into everything we do and helps us meet the worst that life can throw at us with new courage. The book is based on MBCT and focuses on promoting joy and peace rather than banishing unhappiness. It is precisely focused to help people to boost their happiness and confidence levels whilst also reducing anxiety, stress and irritability.

Search Inside Yourself: Increase Productivity, Creativity and Happiness Chade-Meng Tan *Collins*

Chade-Meng Tan's book concerns the mindfulness programme created for Google by a diverse group of individuals including a Zen master, a CEO, a Stanford University scientist and the well-known author Daniel Goleman. The book outlines a personal growth programme that focuses on developing emotional intelligence through mindfulness, to make us more productive at work and better leaders, whilst we are becoming more peaceful, happy and compassionate individuals. It shows us how to apply mindfulness to ourselves, our business and everyday life. Whether we are a junior team member or a senior manager, a secondary school teacher or bus driver, mindfulness has the potential to dramatically improve our life.

The Emotional Life of Your Brain Richard Davidson and Sharon Begley *Hodder & Stoughton*

This groundbreaking book offers a totally new understanding of our emotions – why each of us responds so differently to the same life events, and what we can do to change and improve our emotional lives. From thirty years of studying brain chemistry, Davidson shows how and why we are all so different. Just as we all have our own DNA, so we each have our own emotional "style", depending on how strong our characteristics like resilience, attention and self-awareness may be. By helping us to recognize our own emotional style, Davidson also shows how our brain patterns can change over the course of our lives. The book, illustrated by fascinating experiments, shows what we can do to improve our emotional responses through mindfulness meditation (among other techniques).

Deepening our understanding of the mind–body connection, as well as conditions like autism and depression, Davidson and Begley go beyond mainstream psychology and neuroscience and expands our view of what it means to be human. If you always wanted to know how you tick, this is your book.

A Mindful Nation: How a Simple Practice Can Help Us Reduce Stress, Improve Performance and Recapture the American Spirit Tim Ryan *Hay House*

US politician Ryan here connects the dots for us between what's happening with mindfulness in the classrooms, hospitals, boardrooms, research labs and army bases across the world by sharing his interactions with experts in education, defence, health care, criminal justice and the environment. Both inspiring and pragmatic, the book shows us how we might apply the benefits of mindfulness to the current challenges that affect each of us in our own lives and communities and the implications for our society as a whole.

With a proper understanding of politics, government budgets and what it takes to get something done, Ryan connects a practical approach with a vision of how mindfulness can reinvigorate our core values and transforms and revitalize our communities.

Real-life experience

Reading a book is one thing: it may be inspiring, may nourish our curiosity and so on. But to experience mindfulness we *have* to practise it. The classic way, and one we would recommend after reading this book, is to look for an introductory day or workshop to get a first real-life experience of practising mindfulness.

It may be that you will find that mindfulness is not your cup of tea. On the other hand, if this experience confirms a growing feeling that you should be reading this newly found path, the next leg would be to enrol onto an eight-week programme.

To reap the full benefits of mindfulness – as we hope you will have learned by now – we have to develop our own personal mindfulness practice (both formal and informal). It is always a good idea to seek the help of a "task force" (see p.219). A local "sangha", for example: a mindfulness meditation practice group of like-minded people, with whom you can share the practice and life experience.

To deepen your practice sustainably, it is advisable to participate in mindfulness retreats. There are many providers at many different venues that offer these "away days" from stress and pressure – whether they are under the tropical sun or in the rural surrounding of England's hills and lakes. Some venues are very spartan, others are rustic; some are more stylish and some are even rather posh. Whatever fits your individual style, preference or standard, if you search carefully, you will find your own very special and supportive place.

But it's also possible for us to have a retreat day on our own – at home! Here's an idea of how this could work.

Sample timeline for a personal mindfulness retreat day

6:30	Wake up, shower, dress (informal practice)
7:00	Sit and check-in to mindfulness of breathing (see also Chapter 6 p.74)
7:45	Eat your breakfast mindfully (see p.125)
8:30	Go for a mindful walk or practise meditative walking
9:15	Check-in for a guided body scan meditation (see also Chapter 6 p.68)
10:00	Go for a mindful walk or practise meditative walking
11:00	Sit and check-in for the listening meditation (see also Chapter 6 p.77)
12:00	Eat your lunch mindfully
2:00	Go for a mindful walk or practise meditative walking
3:00	Sit and check-in for observing thoughts (see also Chapter 6 p.83)
3.45	Go for a mindful walk or practise meditative walking
4:30	Sit and check-in for choiceless awareness (see p.258)
5:00	Eat your dinner mindfully
6:00	Go for a mindful walk
7:00	Sit and check-in for an observation of an object of your choice (body, breath, sounds or thoughts)
8:00	Go for a mindful walk or practise meditative walking
9:00	Drink – mindfully – a last cup of tea
	...and afterwards, go mindfully to sleep

A one-day personal mindfulness retreat

A solution-revealing insight is not something we can generate on demand. We cannot simply decree: "tomorrow morning at 9am sharp I will have a totally new perspective on this issue in my life". But we can organize the circumstances in which the wisdom from within is likely to arise. Giving ourselves space creates chances.

If we do opt for a personal mindfulness retreat day, we should approach it without any expectations of dramatic incidents; in fact, we should not expect anything special to happen. We should not expect a totally altered mind state (unless, of course, happiness and relaxation are something totally and utterly extraordinary for you).

On the other hand, happiness and relaxation *are* likely to happen, and these create the optimum conditions for insights to occur. The healing that comes from within begins with insights; it could even happen while you are preparing for the retreat. Who knows what new view is just around the corner of the mind?

Being on the lookout for something specific and particular may divert you from seeing something really wonderful. From research we know that our brain has an incredible ability and everlasting capacity to alter itself – it is what scientists term neuroplasticity – and that this occurs every time the opportunity presents itself. A mindfulness retreat is just such an opportunity.

You can construct a mindfulness day for yourself anywhere. You can stay at home, turn off the phone, leave the TV and computer switched off and *don't start* any work-related tasks. We know that it is difficult to be at home and not be seduced into doing things that we feel need to be done. But it is possible.

If you prefer to have a change of scene, you could check-in at a retreat centre that is open to short-term individual guests or rent a hut or caravan on the beach, or even book into a hotel room for a day. The aesthetics and logistics are different but the instructions and the idea are the same. This is what makes this a retreat day. A spa day cultivates our relaxation by responding to our desires. A mindfulness day, however, cultivates our wisdom by not responding at all.

A mindful eating experience

Eating is a most wonderful opportunity to pay attention – because it is so interesting. It involves more than just one sense organ: not only do we see our food but we smell it and taste it and sometimes – if it's crunchy or sizzling – we can hear it.

And, usually, we eat because we are hungry, so our experience is likely to be pleasant. If the retreat we plan for ourselves includes preparing our own food, we choose foods that we enjoy and which are easy to prepare.

If you are preparing your own food, do it slowly, noticing all the movements that go into making the meal. Do not nibble as you prepare: allow yourself to feel the tension of desire and learn something of the mind's ability to accommodate unfulfilled wants.

Sit down with your food for a minute before you begin eating. Look at the food. Smell it. Notice how you begin to salivate. Notice the impulse to start eating. Notice how the mind feels in the moments before pleasurable activity.

And then begin eating – slowly – by putting the spoon or fork down between bites. Imagine that you are tasting *this* food for the very first time. If you have prepared the food yourself you won't be surprised by what is in it, but you can still be enthralled by it. Everything has its unique flavour.

If you are in a retreat centre, or a hotel, it's possible that you might not like the food on offer. In that case you might be interested in how it feels to dislike something; how hard it sometimes is for the mind to accommodate *not* liking even the smallest of things. We can learn a lot about suffering when not liking and resenting is happening, and a lot about the end of suffering when it passes.

Exercise: formal meditative walking

First of all we want to point out that mindful walking and being fully aware of what's going on around you is always a healthy and calming endeavour. There is a choice between going for a mindful walk, or practising *meditative walking as formal practice*, as we will describe below.

To start with, choose a place that is private and unobstructed, where you can walk back and forth. Look for a path of between two and five metres in length.

If you are walking outdoors, it might be appropriate to find a secluded space so that you don't feel it is likely that you will be watched by people (which may lead you to start second-guessing what they may be thinking about what you are doing).

If you are walking indoors, try to find a furniture-free section of a room or an empty hallway, so that your walking can be relaxed and unobstructed.

You don't need to walk in any way that is unusual. No special balance is needed, no special gracefulness – just plain walking. Walk at a slower pace than normal, as slowly and consciously as possible, but, otherwise, quite normally.

Begin your period of practice by standing still for a few moments at one end of your walking path. You may discover that your entire body is an antenna for sensing the world; you will feel warm or cool, hear sounds, observe what's around you and feel your whole body just standing.

Now bring your attention to your body, starting at the top of the head, then moving down through the head, the shoulders, the arms, the torso and legs, and ending by feeling the sensations of your feet on the ground. Allow your attention to rest on the sensations in the soles of the feet.

Start by shifting your body to one side so that most of your weight rests on one leg. Your other leg is now light and can be consciously moved forward. Move your foot through the air, bringing it back to the ground heel first, followed by a smooth rolling motion bringing whole of the sole down to meet the ground. Now place the weight on the other leg and continue this process of:

* shifting your weight
* lifting the foot
* moving
* touching down, heel first
* rolling onto the sole

  ...and so on

During meditative walking, keep your eyes open so that you stay balanced. We often begin with a normal strolling pace and expect that the limited scope of the walk and its repetitive regularity will allow our body to settle into a slower pace. It usually does. This happens because the mind, with fewer stimuli to process, shifts into a lower gear. Probably the greed impulse, ever on the lookout for something new to experience, surrenders when it realizes that we aren't going anywhere.

At a strolling pace, our view is panoramic and descriptive. At a slower pace, the view is more localized and subjective. If we could sub-title the thoughts that accompany walking, they might look like this:

* pressure on feet
* pressure
* pressure disappearing
* pressure reappearing
* pressure shifting
* lightness
* heaviness
* lightness
* heaviness
* lightness
* "hey, now I've got it! now i'm paying attention...
* ... whoops, I've been distracted!"

starting again...

* pressure on feet
* pressure shifting
* lightness
* moving
* heaviness

Our recommendation is that walking slowly is better than quickly because the point of meditative walking is to notice that things change. But the direct experience of mutability can happen while we are strolling just as easily as when we are stepping slowly. So the guide to what speed limit to adopt is simply that you select the speed at which you are most likely to maintain attention.

You can choose how long you'll walk before you begin but try not to look at your watch; if you have a watch timer or alarm function, set it to alert you to the end of the practice period. Indoors, you could set a kitchen timer. Remember that you are walking *just to have the experience of walking* – not to get somewhere, or to finish the "exercise".

Exercise: choiceless awareness meditation

In the body scan we concentrate on our bodily sensations, whereas in the choiceless awareness meditation we witness whatever arises. That may be sounds, feelings and emotions, thoughts or body sensations.

Acknowledge whatever emerges, non-judgementally and hold it in your awareness until it vanishes again. If something different pops into your awareness, that is fine, acknowledge it and hold it in awareness... and so on.

* Make yourself comfortable
* You may lie down, sit or stand
* When you are ready, close your eyes

The only "task" is to be aware of whatever emerges.

15

Destination mindfulness: arrival

Congratulations, you have more or less arrived at the end of this book! As authors we – Susann and Albert – want to express our gratitude to you for travelling with us on this voyage of discovery to find a radically different way to face everyday life. Let's recap a few important principles from earlier chapters to ensure that you derive optimum benefits from the journey before we look forward to the time after our destination has been reached.

We haven't been on some kind of wild voyage into altered states of consciousness, catapulting us into either bliss or madness. To the contrary, by entering onto this path, we have learned the art of quietly observing the organism that we are, moment by moment, day by day, week by week.

In the process, we have discovered details of our own experience, of how mind and body interact, of what the organism (that we are) is all about in its day to day life. Inevitably, we have encountered difficulties along the way, and required patience, kindness and commitment to overcome them.

The importance of practice

Together, we have been working to change patterns of mind that have often been around for a long time – perhaps all your life. These patterns may have become a habit, and as we have seen, these habits die hard. So we have re-learned to use our mind to re-wire the brain and harmonize our relationships. We have understood that we can only expect to succeed in making changes if we put time and effort into learning new skills. After all, the brain needs time to rewire.

Please use the resources offered in this guide and in the downloadable audio exercises to support you in this process. The mindful approach depends entirely on our willingness to practise daily. It involves practising a particular kind of awareness which we slowly hone and deepen over time, perhaps with the help of a teacher – but one chosen very consciously.

We appreciate that it is often very difficult to carve out the necessary time for something new in lives that are already very busy and crowded. However, the commitment to spend time on simply *being* is an essential part of personal practice. Begin slowly – maybe only a few minutes per day – but gradually increase the time spent to whatever works for you.

Facing difficulties

Over time, we become more aware and more *present* in each moment of our life. The good news is that this makes life more interesting, vivid and fulfilling. On the other hand, it means facing what is present, even when it is unpleasant and difficult. As your practice deepens, you will find that, in the long run, turning to face and acknowledge difficulties is the most effective way to reduce unhappiness. Seeing unpleasant feelings, thoughts or experiences clearly, as they arise, means that we will be in much better shape to nip them in the bud before they worsen into more intense or persistent ill health.

Through mindfulness practice we will develop gentle ways to face difficulties. We can also find guidance from a teacher and support from other like-minded people of the mindfulness community.

Patience and persistence

The effects of our effort usually only become apparent over time. In many ways it is much like gardening – we have to prepare the ground, plant the seeds, ensure that they are adequately watered and nourished, weed the patch and then wait patiently for results.

We must *consciously* progress on our journey and do so with a spirit of patience and persistence, committing ourselves to putting time and effort into our practice, while accepting with patience that the fruits of our efforts may not show straight away.

The future of mindfulness

As we have seen, mindfulness is now being used in schools, universities, diverse workplaces, medicine, therapy and even prisons. Mindfulness is regularly in the news and ever more widely researched. We have Jon Kabat-Zinn to thank for a great deal of this. Although some newspapers portray mindfulness as a passing fad, we agree with Jon that "a text book has not been written on what's possible". Neuroscience – especially the field of neuro-plasticity – is starting to prove mindfulness' potential already.

Until fairly recently science regarded the brain as largely immutable and fixed. We are now discovering that the brain has the capability to change by re-wiring itself through the power of thought. Mindfulness helps us recognize our thoughts and choose how we respond to them, rather than reacting on autopilot. In effect we change our mind to change our brain to change our mind. The possibilities for self-development and wellbeing are limitless.

As Jon said in June 2012 during a training retreat in Salzburg: "integrating mindfulness into society is not the job of the Dalai Lama – it's not up to me, it's up to you".

We, the authors – as part of the mindfulness community – would be delighted if you chose to stick with us on this once-in-a-lifetime, fascinating journey: travelling from the nightmare of a life on automatic pilot to one designed according to your own vision. Stay mindful and fare well.

Index

A

N